ACUPUNCTURE
A Patient's Guide

An introductory guide, using western scientific explanations, which describes acupuncture therapy in all its aspects in language a lay reader can easily understand.

✔ **KU-245-180**

ACUPUNCTURE
A Patient's Guide

by

Dr Paul Marcus

M.D., Dip. Pharm. Med.

THORSONS PUBLISHING GROUP
Wellingborough, Northamptonshire

Rochester, Vermont

First published 1984
Second Impression 1987

© PAUL MARCUS 1984

British Library Cataloguing in Publication Data

Marcus, Paul
   Acupuncture
   1. Acupuncture
   I. Title
   615.8'92   RM184
   ISBN 0-7225-0921-9

Printed and bound in Great Britain

Contents

Introduction

I have practised acupuncture for ten years or so, and have seen a tremendous change in the attitudes of the public and the medical profession to this form of medicine over that time. At first there was widespread ignorance amongst lay people; whereas doctors, if they knew about acupuncture at all, generally dismissed it as a form of hypnosis or suggestion at best, or charlatanism at worst. Quite rapidly as changes in medicine go, knowledge of this therapy has spread widely throughout the United Kingdom. The attitude of most of the profession has become much more open; a sentiment of 'let's see what it can do', with a number of doctors using acupuncture enthusiastically in their everyday practice.

The cause of this transformation is easy to find: it is the enormous amount of publicity which acupuncture has received, both in the public media: newspapers, magazines, radio and television, and in learned journals which present medical case reports and the results of clinical trials. There are two reasons for this dramatic publicity. The first is that acupuncture is a somewhat bizarre form of treatment, exciting considerable interest because of the way in which it is administered. The second is: it works! As Aldous Huxley wrote: 'that a needle stuck into the skin of the foot should help a case of migraine is obviously incredible; it makes no sense. Within our system of explanation there is no reason why the needle prick should be followed by an improvement. Therefore we say it cannot happen. The only trouble with this argument is that as a matter of empirical fact, it does happen'.

Despite the upsurge in interest in acupuncture there is still considerable ignorance, and many misconceptions about it are prevalent amongst doctors and patients. Doctors are fairly well served by textbooks and balanced, objective surveys of the indications for the method and its capabilities, which have been published in the literature. There are now excellent courses of instruction available, which do not necessitate the doctor having to travel to China, and most surgical instrument manufacturers carry a range of the equipment necessary for practising the technique. But the patient is much worse off. He needs to know what can be expected from acupuncture, which conditions it will benefit, where it can be obtained and whether there are side-effects or other problems associated with it. In short he requires a guidebook to help in negotiating this largely uncharted country; because there are many hazards and pitfalls.

Over the time I have spent in treating a variety of different patients with acupuncture, certain questions have been asked again and again. This book is a considerable expansion of a sheet of notes which explains the most important points about acupuncture, which I give to patients in my practice. Of course, it needs to be much longer than the notes since the reader relies only on the written word, and does not have an acupuncturist available to explain anything which is not immediately clear. I believe that as doctors we have somewhat forgotten the art of communicating to patients, whilst advancing marvellously in technical matters. A full explanation of the expected course of events, the risk of complications, and so on, does much to avoid problems associated with any form of treatment, and to enhance the possibility of cure. This is clearly of the utmost importance with a form of therapy which is still largely shrouded in mystery, so the patient does not know what to expect.

The book has an essentially practical structure. The first part (Chapters 1 to 5) deals in turn with the queries which will inevitably crop up in the mind of any patient contemplating and undergoing treatment with acupuncture. The second (Chapters 6 and 7) is a brief account of the history of acupuncture, and a partial explanation of its mechanism of action. The explanation is of necessity only partial, because as yet we by no means fully understand how the remarkable benefits acupuncture produces come about. Finally, Chapter 8 is a series of case reports of typical patients treated successfully with acupuncture.

Chapter 1

Why Acupuncture?

Acupuncture has become extremely popular recently, and particularly so in the past five years. Use of this method of treatment has always lagged behind in the United Kingdom compared to other countries in Europe (and, of course, in the Far East), but now many National Health Service general practitioners use it for some of their patients; it is available from full time private medical and non-medical acupuncturists; and anaesthetists and other pain relief specialists include it in their armamentarium for treating chronic pain on an 'in-' or 'out-patient' basis. Also specialists in orthopaedics, rheumatology and sports medicine use acupuncture to provide rapid, safe relief from stiffness, pain and muscle spasm; and obstetricians and midwives use it to relieve the pain of labour. One can hardly pick up a copy of a women's magazine, or turn on the TV set without seeing some new revelation about acupuncture; and lectures for lay or professional people on the subject are characteristically filled to overflowing.

Success and Failure in Modern Medicine

I am sure that one reason for the enormous interest that acupuncture generates is a general dissatisfaction with conventional medicine. We have made wonderful advances in so many areas in the years since the second world war: in antibiotics; organ transplantation; open heart surgery; the treatment of malignant disease; the eradication of smallpox; and yet as a whole we are not satisfied. Why this might be is a very complex question. Some point to the side-effects of treatment; the thalidomide and practolol disasters, the risk of immunization causing neurological illness in children, the high mortality rates of some surgical operations. Others blame the continued restriction of our capabilities despite the investment of huge sums of money and millions of man hours of effort. Thus we have made little impact in reducing the mortality from many common malignancies; strokes and heart disease kill thousands yearly; we cannot halt the inexorable deterioration in senile dementia; we often cannot provide effective treatment for migraine, or backache; we cannot even cure the common cold (although this situation seems likely to change in the near future).

It is undoubtedly true that many common illnesses, which cause the loss of millions of man hours from work and give rise to untold misery to the sufferers, cannot adequately be treated by the conventional methods which are available. We may take backache as an example. It has been estimated that 50 per cent of the population will have suffered a significant degree of back pain by the age of 60. In a substantial proportion of these the pain will be severe, often radiating down the course of the sciatic nerve into the leg and foot (sciatica). Recurrence is extremely common and, in a few unfortunate cases, chronic or permanent disability results. The back is a very complex structure; a series of small joints between adjacent pieces of bone, surrounded by nerves, blood vessels, ligaments and muscles (see Figure 1). The whole system has to support the full weight of the trunk, yet it must retain the flexibility required to allow movement in all directions. Many zoologists feel our lumbar vertebral column is not fully adapted to the erect posture which we adopted in the course of our development from the apes. It is hardly surprising that this weak link in our anatomy malfunctions; nor is it surprising that our knowledge of the cause of the problem is far from precise. Often the reason is a rupture or 'prolapse' of the intervertebral disc of fibrous material between adjacent bones;

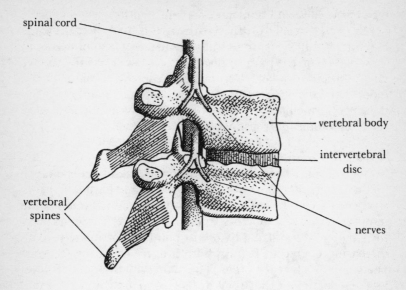

Figure 1. The Spinal Column

but muscles and ligaments can be involved and there are other rarer, but more serious, causes such as tumours or infections of the bones.

Where a cause can be discerned, treatment can be directed towards remedying it; but accurate diagnosis is often impossible and the general term 'low back pain' is frequently used. The standard treatment, particularly for first occurrences and mild attacks, is the prescription of pain killing drugs and/or muscle relaxants, and bed rest on a firm surface, for however long is necessary for the discomfort to go. This commonly takes one to two weeks and often causes severe disruption of the life of an harrassed housewife or busy executive. However, the real problem arises if this treatment fails to produce benefit, or the pain recurs frequently. Then a wide variety of other methods of therapy may be suggested: massage, heat, osteopathy and other forms of manipulation, traction, further bed rest, injections into the spine and, of course, more pain killing drugs. As a last resort, a surgical operation may be carried out. It is a safe bet in medicine that, where a multiplicity of treatments exists for a particular condition, none of them is entirely satisfactory!

Of course, each of these treatments will benefit some patients and it is fortunate that the usual course of events in any case is for the pain to disappear gradually as the tissues heal. But most sufferers from backache will agree that the modern medical practitioner, with all his diagnostic and therapeutic facilities, does not consistently provide relief of their symptoms in a reasonable period of time.

A Lack of Communication

Perhaps in part because of this seeming lack of progress, the quality of the relationship between doctor and patient appears to have changed recently. The old adage that 'in America the patients hate their doctors and in Britain the doctors hate their patients' is starting to lose its point. Unfortunately, to an increasing degree in Britain both are, if not hating, at least being irritated by each other. The main criticism patients level at their doctors is that they do not communicate effectively. They just do not explain what is going on. There rarely seems enough time for the kind word, or the enquiry about the family or hobbies. The patient is not allowed to participate in the discussion, decisions and course of action involved in treating his or her disease, but is made to feel an outsider, baffled by the multiplicity of tests and dazzled by the shiny, stainless steel and visual display units of modern scientific medicine. This reduces the effectiveness of treatment. In fact, as Ivan Illich wrote in *Medical Nemesis*: 'The medical establishment has been a major threat to health.'

The Movement to 'Natural Treatment'

With the growing dissatisfaction in our community with some aspects of mainstream medicine, there has been increasing interest in such things as philosophy, alternative religions, mysticism, more natural ways of eating and fringe medicine. Again, the causes of this are extremely complicated and we should do well to leave discussion of them to the sociologists. Nevertheless it is true that there has been a flood of literature on these matters over the last few years, and they form frequent subjects of debate on the television and radio.

'Alternative' or 'fringe' medicine includes a wide range of different forms of treatment. To be cynical, one may say that they are all characterized by two things: an element of absurdity or bizarreness in the way that they are carried out, and the need for great faith on the part of those who receive them. Thus the patient may be treated by the 'laying on of hands' and asked to believe that some form of vital energy flows from one person to another. Alternatively he may be given a drug or herbal remedy diluted thousands of times more than the concentration which can scientifically be shown to have pharmacological effect. Of course what has been called 'the power of positive prescribing' should not be underestimated. This 'placebo effect' is well known and applies to all forms of medical treatment. A treatment which could not possibly have any intrinsic beneficial action, such as plain water, often produces startling results, even reducing pain or lessening the effect of an asthmatic attack, simply because the patient expects to derive relief from it. The more striking or even outlandish the actual treatment and the circumstances under which it is given, the stronger is the placebo effect usually. Even colour may have a part to play. For example, it has been well known for many years that the ideal colour for anti-rheumatic capsules or tablets is red: they will be found far more effective than white tablets containing the identical drug in the same quantity!

Testing Treatments
Many forms of so-called medical treatment can be shown to be ineffective, and one powerful tool in achieving this is the 'double blind, placebo-controlled' trial utilizing 'random allocation'. Indeed, it is the way governmental drug regulatory authorities in medically sophisticated countries use to demonstrate that new pharmaceutical preparations are sufficiently active to warrant being brought onto the market. The principles of scientific clinical trial design were laid down not very long ago by the famous British Statistician, Austin Bradford Hill. Before then, doctors simply relied on unsubstantiated clinical opinion, now known to be hopelessly unreliable. In a double blind study, neither patient nor doctor

knows which of various alternative treatments the patient is receiving. Therefore neither can be influenced by his expectation of the outcome. 'Placebo-control' implies that one of the forms of treatment that the patient gets is a placebo preparation: a harmless, inactive substance prepared to appear identical to the active drug in every possible way. Lastly, the treatments are allocated at random to different groups of patients, using statistical techniques to ensure that there is no bias in selecting patients for the groups. For instance it would be grossly unfair if most of the patients treated with one method were severely ill, whilst those treated with the other were not so badly affected. The very ill patients would probably do worse than the others just because of the severity of their disease, and not necessarily because of any defect in the treatment.

Why Acupuncture?

Acupuncture certainly qualifies as fringe medicine according to the definition suggested earlier. It is really a very odd form of treatment indeed, involving pushing small needles into the skin at various points, often a long way from the site of the medical problem, and perhaps on the opposite side of the body. On other occasions the traditional acupuncturist may place a small ball of dried herb on a slice of fresh ginger onto the skin, and set light to it! And, as with all such treatments, the patient is required to make an act of faith in accepting the therapy, if only to the extent that he must seek out an acupuncturist and request it. There is no doubt, also, that the association of acupuncture with the Far East increases its popular appeal. Since the days of 'ping pong diplomacy', when the bamboo curtain started to lift, Chinese matters have become of great interest to the public. News that 'barefoot doctors' in rural areas, finding modern drugs next to impossible to obtain, achieve considerable success with acupuncture techniques, certainly satisfies the 'back to nature' enthusiasts and promotes an image of natural medicine without the dangers of side-effects of the artificial chemical drugs which are anathema to this group.

Another characteristic of acupuncture, which probably

accounts for its popularity, is its antiquity. As will be described later, acupuncture probably dates back 5000 years, and there is a tendency at the present to deride modernity and to look to history for acceptable values.

Does it Work?

We have seen that in acupuncture there exists a form of medical treatment which appeals by virtue of its unusual nature, and which has its roots in foreign cultures, ancient times and a more natural environment than that to which Western urban society is subjected. This is true of many paramedical treatments and as was pointed out, many of these, although by no means all, are ineffective. Leaving aside the power of positive prescribing, does acupuncture work? In fact we may reasonably ask, when subjected to double blind, controlled trials can its efficacy be demonstrated? The answer to this question is a qualified yes; qualified because of a number of difficulties any scientific assessor must face. Firstly, although acupuncture is ancient in the East, it has only recently been used and studied extensively in the West. Unfortunately, the latest upsurge of interest has coincided with a period of near bankruptcy for medical research in the UK, and such funds as there are have tended to be diverted to areas of very high priority such as the treatment of cancer and of heart disease. Nonetheless there are active research programmes under way in various European countries, as well as in the East, in America and behind the Iron Curtain. As a result we are learning a good deal about the mechanism of action of acupuncture, a subject which will be dealt with in some detail later.

A technical difficulty arises in setting up controlled trials with acupuncture since it is very hard to devise an acceptable placebo treatment, which is very similar to the active therapy, and yet is itself inactive. For this reason comparisons tend to be made with other standard treatments for the illness in question, such as with analgesic drugs in the management of chronic pain. A further difficulty is lack of organization amongst medical acupuncturists in the West, so that it is hard to assemble a suitably large series of patients with the same

disease for random allocation of treatment by acupuncture
and a comparative technique. Most acupuncturists work in
isolation, seeing relatively small numbers of patients with a
very wide range of medical conditions.

Notwithstanding all these problems some carefully controlled trials have now been carried out, and a steady stream
of reports has appeared in the medical press. Naturally results
have been negative or unclear in some cases, but in general,
the definitive demonstrations of efficacy and safety which have
been made in many different clinical situations have been a
potent force in changing the tide of western medical opinion
from scepticism to acceptance, albeit a cautious acceptance as
yet.

What are its benefits?

This chapter has examined the reasons why acupuncture has
become so popular in the West recently. In that sense it
answers the question posed by its title, 'Why Acupuncture?',
largely by explaining the cultural and philosophical changes
which are leading people to try 'alternative medicine'. But this
book is practical, not philosophical, so the question should
also be answered in a practical way. Actually, most of the rest
of the book explains the kind of benefits, and problems, which
treatment by acupuncture may bring. So the information it
presents may be utilized in forming a sensible decision as to
whether to seek treatment by this method, and how long to
persevere with it.

Suffice it to say at this point that patients should look for
treatment by acupuncture when they have a problem which
has resisted conventional treatment; or where conventional
treatment has serious disadvantages, such as prolonged bed
rest in low back pain; or side-effects, such as the use of a particular drug in an individual allergic to it. Certainly, used
properly, there is little potential for harm in acupuncture, and
improvements are possible in cases which have not responded
to comprehensive prolonged conventional treatment.

These are important benefits indeed, and clearly account
for much of the method's popularity, as do the sociological
changes previously referred to. An additional factor, which

should not be minimized, is the individual attention that patients can expect from most acupuncturists: a willingness to treat the patient as a whole person, to discuss fully the symptoms and other features of the case, and to explain in some detail the nature of the treatment. Of course, this approach is not the sole prerogative of acupuncturists but it is much more likely in private practice than in the frenetic conditions of the National Health Service; and most acupuncturists are private practitioners.

Chapter 2

Will My Condition Benefit from Acupuncture?

This is the very first question any potential patient will require answered. No form of medical treatment is universally applicable, and so it is necessary to decide when to use a treatment and, often more important, when to utilize an alternative technique. In an ideal world it would not be necessary for any lay person to read this chapter, since the decision whether or not to treat an illness by acupuncture would be taken by his medical adviser; usually his general practitioner. Unfortunately, because acupuncture is relatively new in Britain, conventional doctors have not yet fully understood when and how it should be used. Indeed, the intending patient will often be met with a blank look, surprise, or even hostility if he mentions acupuncture to his family doctor. Things are changing rapidly, but still it is necessary for patients to be aware of which illness might be improved by acupuncture so they can actively set about seeking this form of treatment (and how to do this is discussed in detail later in the book), if necessary educating their doctor en route!

Which Illnesses Can Respond?
Until quite recently the only books on acupuncture available in the West dealt with the subject exclusively along traditional Eastern philosophical lines. Many were, in fact, literal translations of ancient Chinese texts. These works showed

enormous therapeutic optimism, stating that acupuncture could be used successfully to treat all known diseases and miraculous results were claimed. Now, the indications for acupuncture are much more clearly understood although, as will be seen, there are still many surprises in store.

The responses of different diseases vary very greatly, and modern Western medical acupuncturists divide them into groups according to the improvement to be expected. Some illnesses such as migraine or trigeminal neuralgia, almost always respond to a worthwhile degree. Others such as rheumatoid arthritis or asthma, only sometimes respond, and the improvement may be only partial. A further group of diseases, such as infections and malignant disease, usually show no improvement at all, although the symptoms they cause may be alleviated. I had considered including here a list of the illnesses which fall into the above three categories, but finally decided that it would not be helpful to do so. There are many hundreds of diseases, and so the list would have been a very long one. But apart from this, there are so many other factors which affect whether or not a given illness will respond in a given individual, that really the only sensible approach for a patient is to go and talk to the expert — the acupuncturist himself! Apart from this, most patients do not accurately know their diagnosis. A person may know he has rheumatoid arthritis, for exmaple, but which form of rheumatoid arthritis, affecting which joints and other organs, and undergoing pre- cisely what form of medical treatment? All of these factors are highly relevant in determining the likely outcome of treatment by acupuncture.

One thing is certainly true, however, and that is it is not good enough for a patient simply to ask his own doctor whether the illness would be likely to respond, unless this doctor happens personally to be very interested in acupuncture. As stated previously, general practitioners and most other conventional doctors are not yet very knowledge- able about this subject and, whilst they will readily think of backache and migraine as candidates for acupuncture because of medical and general publicity about the treatment of these complaints, they are unlikely to recommend the treatment for say naso-sinusitis, in which condition acupuncture often works very well. If I seem to be suggesting that a patient's general practitioner should be excluded from the process of obtaining treatment from an acupuncturist, I'd like to correct that impression at once. As will be seen I feel that the family doctor has a vital part to play, since he takes general medical responsibility for the patient and should decide what is the best form of treatment having regard for all of the patient's personal and medical circumstances. However, the patient too has important rights in the matter, and the whole exercise should be a collaborative one.

Individual Variation

Another complicating factor in the process of deciding whether or not to treat by acupuncture, is the individual variation that occurs. We may take two seemingly identical cases of gastric hyperacidity and dyspepsia. They may be patients of the same age and sex, with identical symptoms, of the same severity and duration, yet one may respond perfectly to acupuncture, and the other not at all. Why this may be is not understood. Nor, in the present state of the art is it predictable in all but a few cases. This difficulty works two ways of course. On the one hand, individual patients with diseases which are usually easy to treat with acupuncture may, unfortunately, not respond. On the other, a few patients with illness usually very resistant to treatment may be considerably benefited. In practice, therefore, when a patient asks an acupuncturist, 'is it worthwhile for someone with my condition to try treatment with acupuncture?' the answer is usually 'yes'. In most diseases there is at least a small chance of response, and of course in many the chances are very good indeed.

All this may sound very confusing, but it reflects a situation which exists during the early stages of the introduction of any novel treatment — a period of discovering, preferably by carefully controlled clinical trials, in which illness the method is useful, and of trying to understand, by scientific research, how the treatment brings about its effects.

Acute and Chronic Illnesses

One thing is clear about acupuncture: other things being equal, it will work more readily in acute rather than chronic disorders. This is common sense. After all, if an illness has a chance to become entrenched, and perhaps to cause considerable damage to the body tissues, it is obviously less likely to respond. It is a pity, therefore, that in modern Western practice, the acupuncturist usually sees patients after they have suffered from their problem for a considerable period and have run through the whole gamut of conventional therapies.

In fact, prevention is better than cure, and traditional oriental acupuncturists were strong advocates of regular treatment to restore slight 'disorders of energy balance' within the body in an attempt to prevent clinical illness becoming manifest. Preventive medicine is expensive, and many would argue that it is not cost effective in the United Kindom, where there are so many high priorities already in treating established disease, so this ideal use of acupuncture in a prophylactic way seems unlikely to come about in the near future.

Is Acupuncture Effective Once Tissue Damage Has Occurred?

The possibility of long-standing illness damaging body tissues was mentioned above. It will come as no surprise to learn that acupuncture is far more effective in treating disorders of tissue function, such as a disorder of nervous system electrical activity which causes chronic pain, than it is in dealing with organic change in some tissue incapable of repairing itself. Once rheumatoid arthritis, for example, has caused muscle wasting and bony resorption leading to deformities of the joints, this process is not reversible by acupuncture; nor indeed by any other medical treatment. However, acupuncture will probably relieve pain and stiffness and even joint swelling in even a severely affected chronic arthritic. On the other hand it is ideally suited to treating the traumatic injury to muscles and joints, which a young sportsman may incur, particularly if it is used soon after the injury.

An important piece of practical advice arises from the above; and that is to seek treatment by acupuncture at the earliest possible time. In fact this advice applies to every other form of medical treatment, for it is much easier to deal with a condition by drugs or surgery as well as by acupuncture early on, perhaps before irreversible damage has occurred.

Biorhythms

One interesting possibility which may affect whether a given patient with a particular disease will respond to treatment concerns the time of day and the day of the month that treatment is given. It has long been known that very many bodily processes are subject to temporal biorhythms. For instance there is a prominent 'circadian rhythm' (i.e., 'about a day' or lasting 24 hours) in such things as the deep temperature of the body and the levels in the blood of minerals and hormones. In women the hormonal axis between the pituitary gland near the brain and the reproductive organs imposes a monthly cycle. Traditional acupuncturists prefer to carry out different forms of treatment at different hours of the day or night, claiming better responses as a result. Other, longer cycles are also described. Whether or not this is true there are few opportunities in the West for treating patients at 'unsocial' hours, and so occasions to test this hypothesis are limited.

Do Other Treatments Affect Response to Acupuncture?

Another complicating factor determining response to treatment is the other forms of treatment which may have been given. Acupuncture works by stimulating the fine nerves in the skin and also, in some cases, deeper organs. Because of this, if the nerve supply has been disrupted, perhaps by surgery or radiotherapy or by a viral infection as in herpes zoster, response to treatment can be unpredictable. At a purely practical level, treatment may be made exceedingly difficult because some surgical procedure has altered the anatomical landmarks which the acupuncturist uses accurately to identify the points for treatment, or by the degree of deformity which exists.

Sometimes treatment with drugs interferes; particularly drugs acting on the nervous system and those that modify the body's inflammatory response. Regarding the former, we know this as a practically observed clinical fact. As I said before, acupuncture works by stimulating the network of fine nerves passing all over the body. These nerves run together and form larger ones. These in turn join to form trunks and finally enter the thick column of nervous tissue which passes up the centre of the spine into the bottom of the brain: the spinal cord. Very many of the drugs which are used in medicine have an effect on the central nervous system. Many are primarily intended for this purpose — such as tranquillizers, hypnotics or antidepressants. Others have this action as a side effect which is not part of their main purpose. Thus antihistamines, which may be used for allergy or travel sickness, often have a depressant effect on the brain and may cause drowsiness. It is to be expected that drugs altering the state of activity of the brain might interfere with acupuncture because, although it stimulates peripheral nerve endings, it must be the cross communication which the nerves make centrally, in the spinal cord and brain, which actually result in the beneficial action of acupuncture being manifest. We do not know how this happens, and we do not know how centrally acting drugs may interfere; but this interference is not a surprising finding.

The way in which anti-inflammatory agents may interfere with acupuncture may not be so immediately obvious. When an acupuncture needle is placed into the skin it causes damage to the tissues through which it passes. The larger and blunter the needle, the more it is manipulated, the longer it is left in, and the deeper it is inserted; the more the tissue damage. Following any damage to the body, the organism sets up a protective response we call 'inflammation'. The blood supply to the area is increased, certain chemical substances are released and scavenging blood cells migrate to the location. The purpose of this response is to combat any infection and to heal the disrupted tissues. One by-product of the release of some of the chemicals involved is an increased sensitivity of the local nerves. The chemicals act on them to reduce the threshold stimulus which causes them to fire electrical impulses towards the brain. In other words they are stimulated more easily. Again this has a protective function, shielding the damaged area from further trauma. It is a common experience that after a cut or burn to the skin even gentle contact with the area causes pain: we say it is 'tender'. After acupuncture, the inflammatory response presumably ensures that nerves that were stimulated by the needle in the first place are constantly restimulated by trivial contact of the skin over the ensuing days. Without this reinforcement the effect of acupuncture would be exceedingly short lived, and it is for this reason that anti-inflammatory drugs are contra-indicated in conjunction with acupuncture. Examples of such drugs are the antihistamines previously mentioned; steroids such as cortisone, used in arthritis and diseases of the immune system; and so called non-steroidal anti-inflammatory drugs such as aspirin and butazolidine.

In many cases in practice the interference with acupuncture caused by these drugs is only partial or does not occur at all. Once again there is enormous individual variation, and the outcome is not possible to predict with any accuracy. Corticosteroids, however, are very powerful anti-inflammatory agents, and in most cases the acupuncturist will wish to avoid treating patients taking these drugs, or may arrange for the drugs to be stopped first. One important point to make here is that steroids should never be stopped abruptly. Serious illness may result until the body's endogenous production of steroids can take over from where the external administration has left off. The dosage of steroid drugs therefore, is always tailed off very gradually.

Fortunately, once drugs acting on the nervous system or those that diminish the body's inflammatory responses are stopped they are usually cleared from the system very rapidly, and then response to acupuncture becomes normal. For this reason previous administration of these agents does not preclude treatment with acupuncture.

Patients often ask whether the fact that they have received many forms of medical treatment in the past makes them unsuitable for acupuncture. They may have had a score of drugs, manipulation, massage, infra red or ultra violet therapy, or a variety of surgical procedures. Apart from the cases mentioned above, there is no particular reason why a multitude of previous therapies should make a patient more difficult to treat; except that this implies that their illness is long-standing and, as stated, chronic diseases are understandably harder to cure than acute ones.

Do I Have to Believe in Acupuncture for it to Work?

I have often been asked by patients whether their psychological state will have any effect on the outcome of the treatment. In my experience, it makes very little difference indeed. Patients who firmly believe that they will be helped by acupuncture, others who have an entrenched resistance to the idea and who have come only to silence a nagging spouse, and those who are indifferent: all seem to have an equal chance of success. Because of the 'placebo effect' referred to elsewhere, it might be thought that acupuncture enthusiasts might be more likely to respond simply due to suggestion. However, suggestibility and placebo effects are less predictable than that. Often it is the person who protests his disbelief the loudest who actually believes most strongly, perhaps at a subconscious level.

Some psychiatric disorders seem to militate against response to acupuncture. Neurotic anxiety and depression seem not to matter and, in fact, can themselves be treated by acupuncture. Psychotic illness, such as schizophrenia, is not only very resistant to acupuncture therapy, but seems to interfere with the treatment of other coexisting illnesses. The same thing applies to persons suffering from a psychopathic personality disorder.

Predicting Response

It will be seen that providing an answer to the one question every patient wishes to ask, 'will my condition benefit?' is *exceedingly* difficult in the individual case. The response of different diseases varies greatly and so does the response of individual patients with the same disease. Concurrent drug treatment may interfere, biorhythms may be important and there is certainly a large number of factors which influence response which we do not even know about. As time passes, more and more patients will be treated with acupuncture under controlled conditions and the results collected and published as 'series' of cases of particular diseases. Then it will be possible, by reference to the medical literature, to determine what proportion of persons with a particular illness can be expected to respond to treatment. Thus, we may say that in trigeminal neuralgia the response rate is 80 per cent. This means that, if we take 100 patients with this condition (which causes severe pain in the side of the face) and treat them with acupuncture, using the correct points and for long enough, probably 80 of them will respond. If we consider any given patient, we do not know in advance whether he or she will benefit from the treatment; we can only say that there is an 80 per cent chance of them doing so.

There are many difficulties in assessing response data of this kind. For instance, the definition of response must be precise. Does the author of the paper mean *any* relief of pain however slight or transient; only relief which the patient or his doctor considers worthwhile; or what? Specialist medical acupuncturists are, of course, intensely interested in these matters and are likely to have the most up to date information on how effective their treatments are. The general medical practitioner is less likely to be knowledgeable, because his sphere of interest encompasses almost the whole of medicine. However, for very many reasons it is essential for an intending acupuncture patient to involve his GP in obtaining treatment (more about this later). So he should ask the above all important question of his GP first of all; but should not be easily discouraged from speaking personally to the acupuncturist who might treat him. Even this 'expert' will give an answer couched in terms of probabilities and possibilities, rather than firm, confident predictions.

So, in the last analysis it is the patient himself who must evaluate the equation, balancing the chances of success, so far as they can be determined, against cost, inconvenience and the possibilities of adverse events resulting from the treatment. In very many cases, and particularly those in which the patient has suffered discomfort for long periods and in which a safe, convenient and highly effective conventional remedy is not readily available, the answer will be 'give acupuncture a try'. In many diseases the possibilities of relief are very high. In nearly every one there is some chance of success, and, as we shall see, the likelihood of adverse consequences arising from the treatment is extremely slight, providing the treatment is carried out with normal medical standards of care.

Chapter 3

How Can I Find An Acupuncturist?

The mechanics of acupuncture are extremely simple. It does not necessitate years of training or practice to push a fine needle into the skin, or to massage certain points, or to treat by cautery. The equipment needed for treatments is now freely available in the United Kingdom from surgical instrument manufacturers, or even oriental bookshops. What does, of course, require considerable skill and training is the choice of points and methods of treatment which are appropriate to the particular condition and the individual patient being treated. Unfortunately it is not easy for a patient to know whether a practitioner is being skilful, and so the correct selection of a person to carry out the therapy is critically important.

In Britain there is no legal reason why any individual should not at once call himself an acupuncturist and set up a practice for the treatment of patients. Indeed, apart from members of the main acupunture associations there are far fewer restrictions placed upon the lay acupuncturist than on the medically qualified one. For these reasons, there is every opportunity for untrained persons to practice acupuncture. Since there are certain dangers inherent in the process of treatment by acupuncture, this is a very unsatisfactory state of affairs; which I wish to examine in more detail.

When a person after five or six years of study at medical

school, qualifies as a medical practitioner in the UK, he must carry out not less than one year in recognized hospital appointments, one in a medical speciality, one in a surgical one. Following this, if his performance has been satisfactory, he can apply to the General Medical Council for acceptance as a 'Registered Medical Practitioner'. It would take a lot of space to list all of the subjects studied during a doctor's training period. They include, of course: anatomy, bacteriology and the diagnosis of disease, as well as a wide variety of methods of treatment. (There are many who say that the undergraduate medical syllabus is far too crowded.) At each stage of the process the candidate is carefully examined to see that his standard of competence achieves acceptable levels.

Following registration, the medical practitioner can work in any branch of medicine, and must undergo further prolonged training before achieving specialist qualifications in, say, surgery, psychiatry or cardiology. Recently a three-year period of compulsory postgraduate training for general practitioners too has been introduced. The specialist does not normally see patients directly, but has them referred to him from a general practitioner; a situation analogous to that which exists between barrister and solicitor. The virtue of this arrangement, which is sometimes criticized by patients and their organizations, is that a G.P., with his broad knowledge of medicine, can assess the patient's illness and direct him toward the most appropriate specialization. Additionally, knowledge of the patient's personal and social background allows him to act in the capacity of friend, filtering and advice of the specialist, who may not have such a long-standing acquaintance with the patient, and making sure it is fully appropriate to his family and business circumstances and needs as an individual.

Registration with the General Medical Council imposes a number of constraints on the doctor: a few benefits and not a few disadvantages! There is a comprehensive code of practice for the medical profession, as with other professions, and one aspect of this concerns the prohibition of advertising. Unlike in some countries, in Britain medical practitioners may not advertise their services, either to their patients or to other doctors who might send patients to them. There are very sensible reasons for specialists not advertising to the public. The benefits of the patient should be paramount, and not the size of the doctor's list. Patients themselves cannot easily judge the relative competence of a doctor; whereas one doctor will readily form an opinion of another.

Therefore the accepted procedure in Britain is always for one doctor (the general practitioner) to refer patients to another (the specialist). This system can be criticized, and is at its worst in respect of rather new specialities such as acupuncture, pain relief or perhaps oncology (the treatment of cancer), which are not fully understood by some general practitioners. In these areas, and some others, more direct contact between patient and specialist might be beneficial, if only because it is the specialist alone who possesses all the most up to date facts about which conditions may respond to his particular treatment, what are the contra-indications, and so on. Another serious objection to a specialist's inability to advertise is that many lay practitioners are completely unrestricted. For instance, an acupuncturist who is not a member of the main acupuncture associations and included in the Register of British Acupuncturists (who are subject to virtually the same restraints as a registered medical practitioner with regard to advertising and ethical conduct) could put his name up in neon lights outside his clinic, could hand out in the street sheets describing the benefits of his treatment, and could even take a full page advertisement in the local paper. Of course, it is also true to say that such unregistered lay acupuncturists suffer from one important disadvantage: many medical practitioners will not refer patients to them.

As suggested there are very many lay practitioners of acupuncture who are well trained and operate to the highest ethical standards. They undergo prolonged training in reputable schools and are carefully assessed before being allowed to practise. They see hundreds of patients each year and, as time goes by, amass a large store of practical experience which allows them to treat successfully many different medical conditions. The other side of the coin is that inevitably some qualified doctors using acupuncture will have less extensive experience, simply because this method of treatment is relatively new to British medicine. Furthermore, one considerable advantage to the patient in obtaining treatment from the non-medical acupuncturist is that he can easily find one, probably only a short distance from where he lives, and he can ring for an appointment without the sometimes lengthy process of asking his general practitioner to refer him, which many patients feel rather diffident about.

The Medical Referral

Does it matter then whether a patient receives acupuncture from a doctor or from a lay person, who may have studied acupuncture as carefully, or more so, and for a long or longer time than the registered medical practitioner? I believe personally that the answer to this question is: yes, for a number of reasons. The first is that referral by a general practitioner, or from one specialist to another, is actually very important. The first doctor will send a letter to his colleague summarizing his diagnosis, any tests carried out to establish this, and the kinds of treatment which have been used in the past. Current treatment will also be explained; a matter of great importance in determining the response to acupuncture (see Chapter 2). He will be available to consult with the medical acupuncturist about some detail which is perhaps not clear, and he will receive frequent reports from the latter during the treatment process and when treatment is over so he can arrange for any follow up procedures the specialist advises.

Another major advantage in attending a medically qualified acupuncturist is his training in diagnosis. Naturally, when a general practitioner sends a patient for treatment, he will explain the diagnosis fully to the specialist, but this doctor will also examine the patient carefully and may require further X-rays or laboratory examinations to be carried out (which would be difficult or even impossible for the lay acupuncturist to arrange, even if he could interpret them). Based on his findings he will form his own opinion as to the diagnosis (a 'second opinion' in fact), and this process is clearly beneficial to the patient. Apart from this, medical conditions change with time, and the specialist can keep watch on an illness during the period the patient is in his care, and may detect new signs, or even a totally new condition developing. At any time the acupuncture specialist feels it is advisable, he can refer the patient to another specialist colleague, such as an orthopaedic surgeon, a general physician or a neurologist. Or he may simply request a consultant opinion on a particular aspect of the case, retaining the overall care of the patient for the time being.

A further advantage in obtaining acupuncture from a qualified doctor is that he is not restricted to this form of treatment but can change to conventional medicine at any time, or combine the two. For instance, he may prescribe pain-killing drugs in the early stages of treatment of a case of lumbago, tailing them off gradually as the patient's pain begins to respond to acupuncture. He can also, in consultation with the patient's general practitioner, reduce or otherwise modify treatments the doctor had previously prescribed.

Lastly, acupuncture is not totally without hazard, particularly if misused. We shall explore this subject in much more detail later; but for the present, it will be clear that if a needle is inserted into the body there is potential for damaging important structures under the skin, such as nerves or blood vessels, and for introducing infection. Some body areas are particularly susceptible to infections, such as the cavities of joints. If bacteria enter joints, they may set up a septic condition which can eventually lead to arthritis; and the areas of skin around joints are often the subject of attention by acupuncturists.

Another particularly dangerous infection is hepatitis, which can be passed from one patient to another if needles and other instruments are improperly sterilized. Boiling is not adequate in this respect and disposable needles must be used, sterilized by irradiation, or the instruments should be treated by autoclaving or a 'hot air' method. Adequate cleansing of the skin is also advisable. Medical practitioners' experience in anatomy teaches them in considerable detail the location of various bodily organs, so they can avoid them in the process of treatment by acupuncture, and training in bacteriology, hygiene and infectious disease provides the knowledge to allow them to avoid the risks of infection during treatment. The best training courses for lay acupuncturists also include this kind of information, which is absolutely essential for them to treat people safely. However, having said this, the main lay associations of acupuncture count among their members a number of doctors and dentists, and there is liaison between lay acupuncturists and medically qualified ones.

Contacting an Acupuncturist

For all of the above reasons I believe that the patient wishing for treatment by acupuncture would do well to ensure that the person that he consults is medically qualified. But actually finding a medical acupuncturist can be very difficult. As stated, general practitioners have little experience of this area and, as yet, few hospitals include treatment by acupuncture amongst their services. The key to this process is again the general practitioner. Even if he has never received the request before, and has no knowledge of a medical acupuncturist in his area, he has access to organizations such as the British Medical Association, and the British Medical Acupuncture Society which maintains lists of practitioners sorted according to geographical area. Alternatively, he can speak to colleagues in general practice or hospital, such as neurologists or anaesthetists, who may have more experience of the subject. Medical practice works largely by a process of personal recommendation by doctors, and specialists who produce good results in a friendly but expert manner soon become known to their peers.

Of course, patients also make personal recommendations. What should a patient do if a friend or relative suggests a particular doctor who has helped them? Well, there is no reason why they should not personally contact the acupuncturist for an informal discussion of their condition, perhaps over the telephone. He will often be able to give a good idea of whether he thinks treatment worthwhile even without hearing from the patient's general practitioner, taking a full medical history or performing an examination. At any rate, he can indicate whether he feels it is worth proceeding to what will be an obligatory next stage: referral by a general practitioner.

Alternatively, the patient can see his doctor first, explain that he has been recommended to see a particular acupuncturist and request referral.

Whichever method by which referral to the accupuncturist comes about, the next stage will be to make an appointment – usually by telephoning the doctor's reception staff. This will be a good time to enquire about any special information the doctor may need during the first consultation. Perhaps the patient may have his own X-ray films, and can bring them with him. He should also bring all the medicines that he is taking currently, for ease of identification. The patient can ask about the location of the surgery, and how long the first appointment will take, and should also determine the acupuncturists's scale of fees.

Chapter 4

What Can I Expect When I'm Treated?

A consultation with a medical acupuncturist is much like one with any other doctor in that it will be made up of three parts: history, examination and treatment. This is the sequence followed by medical practitioners since antiquity. The acupuncturist will first read the letter of referral from the general practitioner who sent the patient to him, and will obtain from this a broad outline of the case. As explained previously, this letter will give a short summary of the primary and secondary conditions, the results of any investigations carried out and the treatment used currently and in the past. This letter is thus a valuable introduction to the problem for the acupuncturist, although it is not actually essential. A telephone conversation may take its place; and sometimes, particularly if the case is a simple one, a patient may be referred without any communication at all. Naturally, in this event, the acupuncturist will have to elicit even the most basic details of the case himself.

Which Questions Will be Asked?
After reading the referral letter the acupuncturist will ask a large number of questions, both specific and general. Some will seem relevant and understandable, and some will appear incomprehensibly irrelevant. They will include many conventional medical enquiries such as: 'Where is the pain? Are

you short of breath? What is your appetite like at present?'
and so on. In this phase of the consultation the acupuncturist
will usually first ask in some detail about the actual symptoms
of which the patient is complaining. He will aim to find out
how long they have been present; their frequency and intensity; whether they are getting worse and, if so, over what time
period; if anything improves or exacerbates them; and how
they impact on aspects of daily life such as eating, sleeping
and working. He will enquire as to the past medical history to
chart important events such as severe illnesses, operations or
stays in hospital. An obstetrical history may be relevant. Next
he will ask a variety of rather general medical questions in the
so-called 'systematic enquiry', designed to draw attention to
problems in body systems other than the one primarily
affected. Shortness of breath and ankle swelling may indicate
a cardiac problem which should be investigated, or a cough
productive of sputum may draw attention to a respiratory condition. The acupuncturist will ask about the health of the
patient's immediate family, since some illnesses are predis-
posed to genetically. He will also enquire about the patient's
social habits, particularly alcohol and tobacco consumption
and how much exercise he takes, because of the influence
these factors have on the state of good or ill-health.

After this conventional medical history has been taken, the
acupuncturist will ask some questions which are specifically
relevant to acupuncture. These will be particularly concerned
with areas of tenderness on the body's surface, which often
assist in diagnosis and may also be important points to treat,
by massage or insertion of needles. The way in which the tenderness in these spots may be caused will be dealt with later.
For instance, it is very common for sufferers from migraine to
complain spontaneously of tenderness of certain localized
points around the back of the neck and tops of the shoulders
(see Figure 2). This may precede the headache, and may be
present for hours or even days afterwards. Similar 'trigger
spots' occur over the lower back, buttocks and legs in cases of
lumbago and sciatica.

Other matters related to acupuncture treatment will be
enquired about at this time, such as the drugs which are being

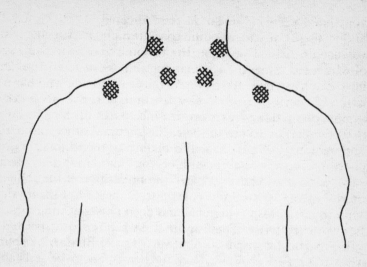

Figure 2. Common trigger spots on the neck and shoulders in migraine.

taken and which may interfere with treatment. If acupuncture has been tried before, the points which were used and the outcome of the treatment are obviously very important.

How Will I Be Examined?

After the history has been taken, the acupuncturist will carry out an examination. Again, this can be sub-divided into parts which are the same as any medical examination, and those which are peculiar to acupuncture. The usual clinical examination will include a careful check of the area which is affected by the illness complained of and also a more rapid routine assessment of all other bodily systems. Many acupuncturists will take the opportunity to check the patient's blood pressure and to look for sugar and protein in the urine, even if there is no reason to suspect that problems in these areas exist. This is a sensible precaution because there is considerable value in detecting, as early as possible, hypertension, or the various illnesses characterized by changes in the constitution of the urine. In female patients, examination of the breasts and a cervical smear may be indicated.

The form of the examination which is specific to acupuncture will depend on the training and beliefs of the acupuncturist himself. The patient will see a considerable difference between a classical practitioner and one who has a more Western attitude. For instance, the traditional acupuncturist sets great store by the 'pulse diagnosis' and may even carry this out to the exclusion of all other forms of examination. The patient will probably be asked to sit with his arms resting on a cushion on his lap whilst the acupuncturist carefully palpates the pulsations of the radial arteries at the wrists. Advocates of this method of diagnosis claim to distinguish superficial and deep pulses at three positions on each wrist. They say that each pulse is associated with a particular organ system, such as the Bladder, Triple Warmer or Pericardium. They further claim to be able to detect almost any bodily dysfunction by changes in the character of the twelve individual pulses, including alterations in energy status which indicate incipient illness, even before it is clinically manifest.

Location of Acupuncture Points

Notwithstanding some differences of opinion between traditionally trained practitioners and those taking a more modern physiological approach, both groups will search carefully for areas of skin which are painful to gentle pressure, for the reasons mentioned before. Even if these are not actually complained of by the patient, they may often be found if looked for, and they are most valuable in indicating particular combinations of points which should be treated.

Time for Discussion

After the patient has had a chance to describe his illness in detail and an examination has been carried out, the acupuncturist will spend some time discussing his assessment of the condition and the role acupuncture may have to play. Of course it may be, at this point, that the acupuncturist will decide that this form of treatment is not appropriate for the particular illness and patient involved. If so, he will say this at the outset and may suggest alternative approaches. He would then return the patient to the referring doctor, sending a letter or telephoning to explain the reasons for his decisions. In many cases, however, he will conclude that the condition is amenable to treatment, and will then probably take some time to explain the form the treatment will take, the number and frequency of the attendances which will be required, and the chances of success. As I have indicated already, individual response is so variable that the acupuncturist can only consider the last two matters very generally, although he will explain that he will be able to judge response much better after the patient has attended two or three times.

The next matter to be discussed will usually be the disadvantages of treatment by acupuncture, and, in particular, the risk of side-effects. This important subject will be dealt with in more depth in the next chapter. It is sufficient to repeat at this point that untoward events are extremely rare when the method is practised by a properly qualified and experienced acupuncturist, and that this almost complete freedom from hazard is one of the major advantages of acupuncture in comparison with conventional therapies.

Actually, any doctor, explaining the possible risk of an intended treatment to his patient, is faced with a considerable dilemma. Absolutely any form of treatment is associated with some risk and, whilst a concerned medical practitioner will wish to present a patient with all the relevant facts to enable him to decide whether treatment should be undertaken, too detailed and comprehensive a description of extremely unusual events will only succeed in engendering unreasonable fear. In some situations a full explanation is essential. An example would be the hazards of a major operative procedure such as open heart surgery, but little would be served by explaining to every patient receiving an aspirin for influenza that there is a tiny risk of a hypersensitivity reaction which could lead to various different rashes, an asthmatic attack, a profound lowering of the blood pressure, indigestion, gastric haemorrhage and the vomiting of blood, and even death! In this situation, as so often in medicine, common sense must be the guide and, since acupuncture is such an inherently safe procedure, the doctor may very reasonably decide not to discuss side-effects in detail unless he is questioned about them.

Can I Ask Questions?

At the conclusion of this discussion, and indeed at any time during the consultation, the patient will be free to ask questions about anything which concerns him, or to ask to have repeated anything which he has not understood. The patient should not be afraid to request an explanation of any points which are unclear. It is not just a matter of satisfying his curiosity; it is actually known that a clear grasp of the aims of the treatment has a beneficial effect in encouraging healing.

When Will the First Treatment be Given?

When all is clear the acupuncturist will suggest that he proceeds to the first treatment, usually then and there, but occasionally at a later date. This may be required for example if it is necessary to tail off some other medical treatment before acupuncture can be commenced, or if further investigations are needed to clarify the diagnosis. Note that, whilst the doctor makes the suggestion, it is for the patient to come to a decision as to whether he wishes to be treated by acupuncture. In making up his mind he will balance the unpleasantness and social disruption caused by the illness, the acupuncturist's advice as to the patient's chances of benefit, and the cost and inconvenience of attending for treatment.

How is Treatment Carried Out?

The aim of all forms of treatment by acupuncture is to stimulate nerves running in the skin, and sometimes in deeper tissues. A small area of inflammation is caused, by mildly damaging the cutaneous tissues, which ensures that the stimulation is long lasting. It follows that any method of causing slight trauma to the skin may be used for acupuncture stimulation, and the acupuncturist will use one or more of these methods depending on the circumstances.

Treatment with Needles and Moxibustion

One of the most common and well-known methods of treating acupuncture points is by using needles. In ancient times these used to be made of ivory or bone, and it is probable that the earliest needles were splinters of hard wood. Next in the historical development of acupuncture, needles of the noble metals were used. Silver and gold will not tarnish, and it used to be thought that needles of these different metals produced different therapeutic effects, 'tonifying' or 'sedating' the system. Most Western trained acupuncturists do not now believe this and needles of fine flexible stainless steel are almost universally used.

Many patients experience considerable trepidation when they are about to receive acupuncture for the first time, and description in the media has much to do with this. Illustrations of acupuncture seem always to show unfortunate patients looking rather like pincushions, with a multiplicity of the largest needles available stuck into them! The photographer often tries to record needles situated in the least pleasant sites too; perhaps the side of the neck or around the eyes. Unfortunately, magazine and TV editors are often less concerned with factual reporting of medical matters than with a sensationalistic presentation with which to improve circulation or viewing figures. In fact it is rare for more than half a dozen acupuncture points to be used at any time, most needles are very short, and of course all areas of the body are treated including the legs, trunk and arms, which are relatively insensitive. The needles used most commonly are about two inches long, half the length being made up of the shaft and half of the handle. However, they are usually only inserted a fraction of an inch into the skin. The shaft has a very sharp point and is made of extremely fine flexible steel (see Figure 3). The handle may simply be smooth, but often has a winding of silver wire to allow the acupuncturist to manipulate it more easily. Silver is chosen for its resistance to corrosion and for its heat conducting properties. For some acupuncture treatments a ball of dried *Artemesia selengensis* (Mugwort or Wormwood) herb may be placed on the top of the needle's handle, when it has been inserted, and set light to. A gentle warmth is then conducted down the needle and this increases the strength of the stimulation. This form of treatment is known as 'moxibustion'. The preparation of the moxa material is a lengthy process. Artemesia leaves are dried and then the veins of each leaf carefully removed. The remainder is ground up with pestle and mortar until a spongy mass, called in China Ai Jong, is obtained. Whether *Artemesia* has any special medicinal properties is debatable, but classical acupuncturists feel that it cannot be substituted by anything else. The modern view is that any form of heat is suitable.

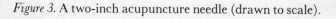

Figure 3. A two-inch acupuncture needle (drawn to scale).

In some forms of acupuncture, now becoming more popular, the needle is inserted more deeply so that its tip contacts the covering of a bone in the area to be treated. This 'periosteal acupuncture' is no more painful than the standard form and is particularly efficacious in some forms of chronic pain. It also has the advantage that fewer needles are required for a given treatment.

Other kinds of needles are also used occasionally; some larger and some smaller. The very long needles, beloved of the Women's Magazines, are occasionally used to treat deep tissues, but more often are inserted parallel to the surface of the body to stimulate several points at once where they lie together in a row. Insertion of these needles causes no more pain than that of the smaller ones. Sometimes a short stubby needle is used and this may have a triangular point. This is employed with a short jabbing movement to raise a minute speck of blood for certain kinds of treatment. This treatment is no more painful than having a vaccination before travelling abroad. Extremely small and fine needles are used to provide a long acting stimulation. They take the form of miniature versions of standard needles, perhaps $\frac{3}{8}$ inch long in total, or whirls of fine wire with a downward facing point, rather like open drawing pins. These are inserted into the superficial layers of the skin and secured in position with surgical tape for days or weeks.

Different acupuncturists have different methods of inserting the needles. Usually the skin will be cleaned with a little alcohol or surgical spirit on a swab and then the point of insertion will be massaged gently with the fingers. The reason for this is to lessen the pain of insertion (in much the same way as rubbing an area which has just been knocked against a hard object reduces the pain). Then the needle is quickly passed into the skin, following the adage: 'Stretch the skin to make it thin and push the needle gently in'. Sometimes numbers of needles are inserted one after the other, the patient is left for a period (usually 15 to 20 minutes) with the needles in situ, and then they are removed. An alternative technique is to use a single needle and to move from point to point, inserting it, manipulating the needle and then removing it. The form of manipulation also varies. Since the handle of the needle is wound with wire, a fingernail run up and down it causes vibration which enhances the stimulation of the point. Alternatively, the needle may be rotated between finger and thumb, and may be alternately withdrawn and advanced at the same time. It used to be thought that different manipulations of the needle caused different effects, but once again, most modern acupuncturists do not adhere to this traditional theory. Now it is believed that the various forms of manipulation only differ in the amount of subcutaneous trauma they cause and, proportionately, in the strength of the stimulation.

Electrical Stimulation

Electrical techniques are used by many practitioners of acupuncture, and especially for pain relief. Certain instruments may be used to detect points for stimulation. Others are utilized to produce an alternating electrical current which is passed down the needle into the skin; and some pieces of equipment can be used in both roles. When instruments are used to locate points, probes are passed over the body and the resistance of the skin is continuously recorded. It is known that acupuncture points are associated with lessened electrical resistance, and so they may be identified in this way. The current may then be passed through the probe or through an electrode which is applied to the skin over the point to be stimulated. This is called transcutaneous electrical nerve stimulation (TENS), and is much used for the treatment of chronic pain by anaesthetists and other pain relief specialists, who may, in fact, use no other form of acupuncture technique. If the trial treatment is successful a patient may be supplied with a portable electrical stimultor which is linked to skin electrodes and he can then alter the intensity and frequency of the stimulation himself until pain relief is maximal, whenever the symptom is experienced.

In another form of electro-acupuncture one or more needles are inserted in the usual way, but they are connected to one output channel of an electrical stimulator. The other channel is then usually connected to an electrode which the patient holds or which is applied to the skin at some non-acupuncture point. Again, an alternating current is passed through the skin, and the frequency, waveform and intensity are adjusted to give maximal benefit. This is analogous to manipulating acupuncture needles manually, but allows more than one point continuously to be stimulated at the same time. It is a particularly necessary adjunct to treatment when acupuncture analgesia for surgical procedures is being induced. In most forms of therapeutic acupuncture transient stimulation is all that is required, but where abolition of the pain of surgery is desired, the stimulation must continue sometime before and during the period of the operation.

Acupuncture During Surgery

Surgical analgesia by acupuncture is little used in Britain and the other developed Western countries. The reason for this is the very high degree of availability, safety and convenience achieved by conventional anaesthetic techniques. This is not the case in all countries of the world and, for instance, there has been a much greater use of acupuncture for this purpose in the Far East. Actually, images of wide awake, smiling patients undergoing major surgery; sipping tea and eating segments of oranges before getting down from the operating table unaided and walking to the ward; have done much to bring acupuncture to the attention of Western doctors and patients alike. Acupuncture is less valuable for abdominal operations in which muscular relaxation is required, although it works well for Caesarian section. It has been used a good deal for surgery of the neck or thorax and for orthopaedic procedures. Even in the West, acupuncture has a place in allowing pain relief during surgery in high risk patients for whom drug-induced anaesthesia might be hazardous, such as the very elderly.

Other Stimulation Techniques

Another method of causing prolonged stimulation is to insert a small thread of suture material into the skin and to knot it into place. This sets up prolonged inflammation, and therefore nerve stimulation, and the effect can be enhanced, when necessary, by the patient tugging the loose end of the thread which projects from the skin. This technique is often used in the treatment of addiction to drugs or cigarettes, or over-consumption of food.

Sometimes injections may be given into the skin. Drugs are not used, but either plain water or concentrated salt solution. The body tissues have a certain normal concentration of salts dissolved in the water in their cells and are said to be 'isotonic'. If they come into close contact with fluids of greatly different tonicity, either hypo- or hyper-tonic, intense irritation is caused. Thus, fluid injections direct into the skin can cause the inflammation which is necessary to treat acupuncture points and, this too, is fairly long lasting.

Yet another way to treat acupuncture points is simply by massage. Firm prolonged pressure or kneading with the fingers or thumbnail will cause a limited cutaneous trauma which can have a therapeutic effect; but this results in a very short lived activity. The major advantage of this form of treatment, however, is that the patient can use it himself. This may be very valuable in some situations. For example, if a patient's illness can be alleviated by acupuncture, but the effect does not last long, it may be possible to teach them the acupuncture points to be stimulated, so that treatment can be carried out at home between visits to the surgery. Alternatively, if it is found necessary to treat a condition at once to abort an attack whilst it is building up, the patient can administer acupuncture to himself at this time by using massage of the points previously found to be effective. It is interesting to note that many of the body areas which are treated by ordinary Western masseurs are rich in acupuncture points, and much of the efficacy of conventional massage certainly depends on acupuncture stimulation.

For treating large areas the acupuncture needle may be lightly grasped midway between the finger and thumb and the point tapped quickly and lightly on to the skin whilst the needle is moved over the part to be treated. Alternatively, the skin can be scratched with the point of the needle, particularly if a line of points is to be treated, such as those running either side of the backbone. Another way of treating a body area is to use what the Chinese charmingly call a 'plum blossom needle' (see Figure 4). This is a small light hammer, nowadays made

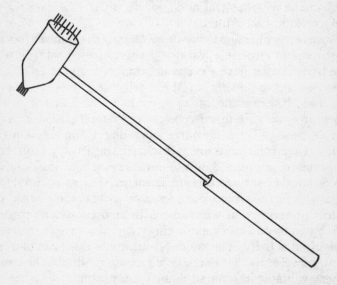

Figure 4. A 'plum blossom' needle.

of plastic, with a double head with fine spikes. On one side the spikes are close together and, when the hammer is tapped on the skin, can be used to treat isolated points. On the other, they are widely separated, and thus lend themselves to stimulating larger areas.

The 'plum blossom needle' is particularly valuable for giving acupuncture treatment to children, who do not mind having their skin tapped, but who usually have a considerable fear of all kinds of needles. Actually, repeated tapping at one position can cause a very powerful stimulation as gradually the superficial skin cells are penetrated and the underlying layers damaged. This is a similar situation to what happens when a badly fitting shoe causes a blister after prolonged walking. The hammer can also be provided to a patient for self-treatment and has the same advantages as with massage, but even greater efficacy.

The only disadvantage is the need to observe scrupulous cleanliness, to avoid the risk of superficial skin infection. Even the needles may be used by patients themselves, but most acupuncturists (and patients) prefer to avoid this situation, unless the patient himself is a doctor or a nurse, because of the chance of wrong insertion and damage to subcutaneous structures. Also, there is a strong, natural, psychological barrier to pushing needles into oneself!

Auriculotherapy

There are two variants of acupuncture which involve treating certain parts of the body only. The traditional acupuncturist, or his modern counterpart, will insert needles at acupuncture loci over all the body; on the trunk, head and neck, limbs, hands and feet. Some practitioners only use the feet, how-ever, (reflexotherapy) and, even more, just the ear (auriculotherapy). Textbooks of these forms of treatment illustrate 'homunculi' superimposed on these organs, showing which positions correspond to the various other parts of the body (see Figure 5). For instance, in asthma, they may obtain excellent therapeutic results by inserting a needle in the precise position on the earlobe which corresponds with the lungs. Other practitioners, the author included, restrict this

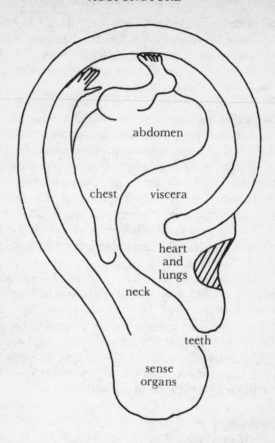

Figure 5. Areas used for treatment by auriculotherapy.

form of treatment to patients who do not respond to the more usual technique involving the whole body; and certainly, in some resistant cases, auriculotherapy is able to give rise to great benefit. Of course, considerable accuracy is required in treating one of so many points in such a small area. One guide in this is to use the tip of the handle of the needle to search for tender points on the lobe of the ear, which often correspond to areas to be treated. In general too, finer needles are used for piqure here than in general body acupuncture.

Heat Treatment

One last form of treatment to be mentioned is cautery. Again, traditional and modern teaching differ. It used to be thought that the treatment of some conditions was better achieved by stimulating certain acupuncture points by heat. Sticks of dried herbs were ignited and held close to the skin; or a cone of herb was placed on to the skin over an acupuncture point and set light to. This latter method could give rise to pain and scarring, of course, and so a variant of the technique was to position a slice of fresh ginger between the cone and the skin. As mentioned, the herb used (*Artemesia*) probably has no special properties except to give rise to a vaguely medicinal smell, and a cigarette can be used in the same way. It is lit and brought close to the skin near an acupuncture point until the patient complains of pain. It is then quickly moved away and the whole process repeated a number of times. Eventually, a red patch of inflammation is caused, which falls short of actual tissue destruction. Many modern Western practitioners of acupuncture feel that there is no particular need to choose this method of stimulating acupuncture points and that results achieved by this means are no different from those from piqure (needling).

How Long Will the Treatment Last?

Patients are, of course, anxious to know how long their course of acupuncture will last. That is, how many treatments will be needed and how long there will be between treatments. It is very hard to give a general answer, as with so many aspects of this subject, because of the tremendous variation in response which occurs between diseases and between individuals with the same disease. As stated, chronic conditions are more difficult to treat and there are certain complicating factors which may interfere with the smooth course of therapy and make repeated treatments necessary. One of the most important factors determining the duration of therapy is how long it takes initially to discover which combination of points will suit a particular patient. As explained, it is rare for more than half a dozen points to be used in combination at any one time, and often only three or four are utilized. Nevertheless, the numbers of possible combinations of the hundreds of points which have so far been discovered in the body run into billions!

Of course, if an acupuncturist relied solely on chance to hit on a successful combination, he would probably take many years to arrive at the best prescription for a patient. Fortunately he is guided by a number of rules which govern how to select the most efficacious points. For instance, points close to the affected area, points at a similar level on the opposite side of the body, points which are tender to the touch, points in areas to which pain radiates, and points close to nerve trunks which supply the affected area, are often indicated to be treated. Also the embryological derivation of tissues is important; that is the way in which the bodily organs develop within the womb. Apart from this, since acupuncture has evolved by a process of trial and error over thousands of years, there is now a large body of experience which can be drawn on. In other words, it has simply been found practically that certain groups of points work in many patients with certain conditions. Even so, the first few sessions of acupuncture are often employed in trying one combination after another until a response occurs, since there is no way to be sure that a given patient will react satisfactorily even to a set of points which benefits most people. Another complicating factor is the strength of treatment which is optimal. Just as with some drugs for which individuals are best suited by smaller or larger doses, so a weak acupuncture treatment may be ineffective or a strong one even counter-productive in some people.

It is for these reasons that acupuncturists will usually wish to wait until the first few treatments have been accomplished before giving confident guidance as to the duration of treatment as well as the chance of benefit.

The Usual Pattern of Response

Assuming a beneficial acupuncture prescription is arrived at it is possible to describe the average course of events for a condition which is not unduly resistant and in which no significant complicating factors exist. Normally, the first session has little or no benefit on the condition being treated. Once again this is not always the case, and, occasionally, lucky individuals may

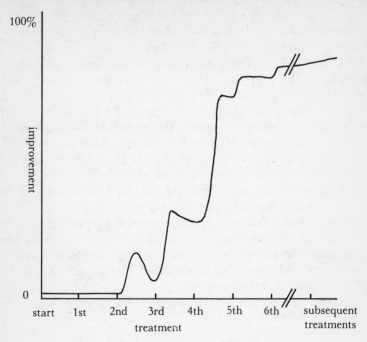

Figure 6. Usual response to acupuncture.

even be totally cured by one treatment. This is rare. The usual course of events is shown in Figure 6. A response is usually noticed after the second treatment and, following the third and fourth, the improvement is rapid. By the fifth or sixth a plateau is being reached and the acupuncturist will start to lengthen the period between consultations. Further, but much slower, progress is then usual, with follow up sessions being carried out over longer periods. Finally, in most patients, a year or eighteen months after the start of treatment no further improvement occurs, but nor does the condition regress even if treatment is stopped. Some patients do require occasional 'top up treatments' for prolonged periods, perhaps every six or twelve months, to prevent their problem returning.

Timing of Treatment

How frequently acupuncture is given during these various

phases depends on a number of factors. Once again, to state the average case, the first five or six treatments will be given weekly. The intervals will then be increased to three to six weeks and then to three months or so. One constraint which influences the frequency of treatment is the frequency with which the symptoms of the patient's illness are experienced. For instance, if a migraine sufferer has a headache nearly every day, the effect of weekly treatments with acupuncture will be easy to judge. If the points have been chosen correctly, after two or three treatments the severity and/or frequency of the attacks will be diminishing. However, a person suffering one severe attack every month may be just as anxious to be rid of the illness. Here it will be necessary to wait several months before a valid judgement of the value of the treatment can be made. Under these circumstances it would be usual for the acupuncturist to see the patient every few weeks and not at longer intervals, since there is evidence to suggest that if the effect of one treatment has completely dissipated before the next one is given there is no 'reinforcement' of one by the other and the eventual outcome is less likely to be successful.

What if there is a Gap in Treatment?

A question patients often ask is whether, during a course of acupuncture, missing a single treatment will undo all the good that has been done. For example, if a patient is midway through a course of weekly treatments and then cannot attend because of holidays or a cold, will this be a severe setback? The answer to this is that usually there is little effect. Of course, the period when the patient did not attend will have been lost from the treatment schedule and eventual completion of the course of therapy will be correspondingly delayed. If the gap is more than a week or so the patient may 'slip back' a little, and need one or two more treatments in total; but there should be little or no effect on the eventual outcome.

How Many Treatments Will I Need?

It will come as no surprise to learn that the total number of treatments required is quite variable. It depends on the disease and severity, the duration of the illness, the frequency with which treatments are given, and, of course, the patient himself. A rough guide for illnesses which respond fairly readily, is that the maximum benefit is obtained initially after six or so treatments, perhaps at weekly intervals. Then two or three 'top ups' will be required at approximately three-monthly intervals, and, finally, one or two more treatments will be needed before the improvement is permanent.

I chose the word 'permanent' at the end of the last paragraph with some trepidation. Naturally, there can be no guarantee that the illness will not recur, and we do not yet have sufficient scientific data following up patients treated successfully, over periods of many years afterwards. There may be various factors which predispose to recurrence. For instance, if there is an anatomical weakness in the back, a sudden wrench or constant overuse may well cause a new attack of pain. But the experience of most acupuncturists suggest that many long-standing symptoms can be relieved for very long periods indeed, and many patients are rid of their complaints for the rest of their lives.

How Long Will Each Session Last?
The duration of each treatment session differs somewhat according to the form the treatment takes and to the amount of discussion and explanation which the acupuncturist includes in the consultation. The first consultation will last thirty to sixty minutes, since it includes the pre-treatment history and clinical examination. During subsequent visits the process will be very much quicker, and the average time taken for the acupuncturist to review progress so far and treat four to six points by simple insertion of needles would be perhaps ten to fifteen minutes. When the practitioner is using acupuncture as part of a Health Service general or hospital practice, there may not be so much time available and there will be a shorter discussion of the problem, the treatment, the chances of success, side-effects and so on. The actual process of treating by acupuncture is extremely straightforward, and can be accomplished rapidly, but most patients (and doctors) feel it is one of the advantages of private medical consultation that time is available for full discussion.

If some less common treatment technique is used, such as moxibustion or electrical stimulation, or if the needles are to be left in situ for some time after insertion for a particular reason, the duration of the treatment itself will be prolonged and even follow-up visits may last twenty to thirty minutes.

What Kind of Benefits Can be Expected?

Symptoms and signs (what is felt by the patient and what can be observed by the doctor) can be reduced in frequency and intensity. They can also change in character to become less troublesome. There may be a reduction in the patient's dependence on drugs or other treatments required to keep their symptoms tolerable. There may also be an improvement in capabilities which have been degraded by the illness, such as the ability to undertake a sport, to carry out a job or to interact socially. All of these benefits may arise at a variety of times after the given treatment.

As stated previously, the first session of acupuncture often seems to do little to improve the situation. Subsequent treatments may then cause benefit, and this will either arise at once, sometimes literally seconds after the insertion of the needles, or within a few days. Further treatments produce greater improvement, and this is less likely to be delayed than that arising after the first session. Finally, when the 'plateau phase' of the primary course of treatment is reached, further treatments have no additional benefit. The reinforcing sessions which are then required because the illness seems to be recurring slightly, will not only restore matters to the status quo but even cause a slightly better state than before. As a result, if the course of the illness under treatment is charted over a period of months or years, there will be seen to be a short lag at the start of treatment, a rapid improvement, a plateau of response and, finally, a very gradual further improvement over a longer time.

It is not uncommon for one symptom of an illness to be more effectively treated than others. For instance, in migraine one of the usual triad of symptons — visual disturbances, nausea, or headache — may respond more rapidly and to a greater degree than the others. Or, to take another example, in osteo-arthritis the pain may be more affected than the stiffness of the joint.

There is an almost infinite number of ways in which acupuncture may affect a given disease in an individual patient, and the best guide to what may be expected will be the acupuncturist himself. This is certainly one of the things about which the patient should ask his doctor before and during the treatment.

What About . . .

Some of the components of normal living clearly influence the response of the illness to treatment by acupuncture and these factors are frequently asked about by patients. Situations influence cases of course, but some general advice is given below. However, the most important dictum, which applies to so many things in life is 'moderation in all things'.

. . . Drugs?

We have already seen that drugs may interfere with acupuncture, and a history of drug consumption will be sought by the doctor. It is very important for the patient to mention any medication he may be taking, even proprietary medicines which may have been purchased over the counter at the pharmacist's shop. Many of these contain powerful drugs which may have undesirable side-effects during treatment with acupuncture. Some of these will have to be reduced in dose or even stopped while treatment is given, but most can be taken as before.

. . . Diet?

Opinion as to the value of special diet in treating medical illness is quite sharply divided. There is no dispute about some clear-cut cases; such as the need for a calorie controlled diet in sugar diabetes, or for a full and varied diet in vitamin deficiency. The dispute comes in respect of a large number of illnesses which have no known direct dietary cause but which many practitioners feel are benefited by diets low or high in fat, protein, carbohydrate, vitamins, minerals, bulk, water and so on. Many acupuncturists have found that their treatment seems generally to work best if a fairly light diet is taken during the therapy period. I usually advise patients simply to 'eat a little less than usual'. Certainly a large meal should be avoided before or just after treatment, and we may speculate (simplistically) that the reason for this is that the body's physiology is then devoted to dealing with the acupuncture stimulus rather than with the absorption, distribution, metabolism and excretion of a large amount of food.

Both conventional acupuncture and auriculotherapy can be used very successfully for the treatment of obesity. They seem to diminish the drive to consume excess amounts of food and are used as an adjunct to a conventional calorie controlled diet. Drug treatment has fallen out of fashion for this purpose, as appetite depressing drugs are associated with many undesirable side-effects, including addiction.

One particularly contentious area is that of so-called food allergies, which have been said to account for a very wide variety of illness. There is even claimed to be a very unfortunate class of patient suffering from 'total allergy' to whom all the substances with which they come into contact in their surroundings, diet and even the air are noxious, but this is outside the realm of acupuncture, and therefore of this book, so I do not propose to examine these possibilities further except to say that, in my view, the case has been rather overstated.

My own philosophy concerning food is to advocate moderate quantities of a good mixed diet. In general it may be safely assumed that if a particular acupuncturist feels that dieting is an important addition to his treatment, he will certainly mention this, and of course his advice should be followed. On the other hand, the patient himself may be a devotee of a particular kind of diet, and this fact must be mentioned to the doctor. Once again the doctor's advice should be followed as restriction or excess of some foodstuffs may be disadvantageous during the period of treatment.

. . . Physical Activity?

We tend to be an overfed and underexercised population in the Western world. If many people would benefit from a moderate reduction of food intake, there is no doubt that many more would do so from a moderate and regular increase in the amount of exercise they undertake. We are not intended to get up from bed, sit on a car or train, sit at a desk, sit again in a car, sit in front of a TV set and get back into bed, day after day. For normal health three or four good sessions of exercise a week are essential. They should last at least half an hour and should make the heart pound, the skin sweat and the chest strain to draw breath. This will improve the muscles, heart, lungs and circulation of a normal person and make disease much less likely at all stages of life. In the case of a person with an existing illness, much the same advice holds, and there are really very few conditions that preclude exercise, provided this is moderate and the patient becomes used to it gradually. Clearly, some diseases affect mobility (such as rheumatoid arthritis) and so prevent some forms of exercise, but others, such as swimming, may often be substituted. The early stages of recuperation from severe infections, heart attacks, strokes and so on are times for rest. But the modern emphasis is very much on a return to activity as soon as possible, and this may not only speed recovery but help prevent further attacks.

As with many such factors, an excess of exercise should be avoided just before treatment with acupuncture and for about six hours afterwards; or the treatment seems less effective. Leaving this aside, the acupuncturist's opinion should be sought as to the best blend of exercise and rest for a particular condition, such as injury to soft tissues occurring during sport, or such as rheumatoid arthritis. It will often be sensible to rest a limb when there is early acute inflammation present but, once this phase is over, progressively to mobilize it to prevent long standing stiffness and even permanent reduction in the range of movement.

. . . Sex?

There is no evidence that sexual intercourse interferes with treatment by acupuncture unless it occurs soon before or afterwards when, like other strong emotional stimuli, it may reduce the effectiveness of some treatments. It would probably be sensible to wait three to six hours after a treatment before having intercourse, for this reason. Occasionally the treatment can itself have effects on the sexual drive in men and women, increasing or diminishing libido. Some acupuncture points are used specifically for this purpose, and the treatment of sexual disorders is an area in which acupuncture can often be extremely valuable. Additionally, sexual activity may be diminished by pain, stiffness, or other symptoms of illness, or sexual interest may be affected by fatigue or anxiety. Then a successful acupuncture treatment, by reducing these influences, may make a sexual relationship more satisfactory.

. . . Alcohol?

It has long been known that excessive consumption of alcohol is undesirable, causing nervous deterioration and toxic effects on the liver. Imbibers will be pleased to learn that it is increasingly evident that moderate consumption may be beneficial, acting as a tension relieving 'safety valve', increasing appetite and even having specific effects in reducing the incidence of some conditions such as coronary heart disease. Excessive consumption of alcohol twenty-four hours before or after treatment by acupuncture undoubtedly reduces the treatment's efficacy, as well as having a general toxic effect on the body, adding a hangover to the patient's other problems. Other than this, a little of what you fancy seems to cause little harm. Certainly wine or beer are much to be preferred to . . .

. . . Smoking?

I fear that the tobacco companies will gain no comfort from me. I feel it is one of the great scandals of modern times that cigarette advertising is still condoned and that the overwhelming weight of evidence linking tobacco use with cancer, bronchitis and heart disease is ignored in many quarters of the government. It seems to me that the advice of any responsible doctor to his patient must be: 'give it up!' Acupuncture is of great value in achieving that. Auriculotherapy seems to be particularly useful in this respect, and a common method of treatment is to insert a small 'press needle' into one of the points on the pinna of the ear, which is then retained for one to three weeks. Alternatively, a suture thread is placed at the same position, which the patient can tug when he feels the urge to light up.

I used to request patients to leave their first cigarette an hour later each day on the principle that a gradual reduction of intake would be less traumatic. With more experience I have now found that there is no substitute for abrupt cessation coinciding with the onset of acupuncture treatment. Support from friends, relations and the spouse is invaluable in this situation, but even so, the incidence of relapse within five years of stopping smoking is depressingly high.

Acupuncture is used for the treatment of addiction to other drugs than those occurring in tobacco smoke, and has achieved notable success in reducing the symptoms of heroin addiction during withdrawal.

How Should I Look After the Site of Treatment?

No special care of the sites of acupuncture is necessary. Washing and bathing can be carried out right away and, in ladies, a small amount of cosmetic applied to conspicuous treatment sites on the face will easily disguise any marks remaining after treatment.

Abnormal swelling, redness, warmth or tenderness at the site of an acupuncture treatment, as well as the discharge of any fluid from the wound, would indicate the presence of local infection, and should be reported to the doctor without delay. This is particularly the case if there are red lines radiating from the puncture site, if there are small painful lumps nearby, or if the patient feels generally unwell with a raised temperature, shivering, headache and other signs of a fever. Infection is exceedingly rare if the proper care is taken towards cleanliness of the skin and acupuncture equipment. I personally have never seen it occur.

Infection is slightly more likely where a needle or suture is left in the skin for long periods. In these cases the onus is on the patient to make sure that the site is kept clean. Once again, tenderness, swelling and so on would indicate a problem and should be reported to the acupuncturist or other doctor as soon as possible.

Chapter 5

What Are The Disadvantages?

It may have been expected that I should deal with the question of the sensations experienced during acupuncture treatment within the previous chapter. However, I find that nearly every patient expects to suffer considerable pain from acupuncture treatment, and this seemed to me to be one of the first points about which an attending sufferer would require reassurance. It would be natural to turn to this part of the book at an early stage, and the question could be answered at this point together with a description of sensation which acupuncture causes.

Let it be said right away, significant pain is extremely rare. The different treatments which are available all have slightly differing sensations associated with them. Moxibustion causes a feeling of warmth passing to very slight discomfort, at which point the acupuncturist will stop the stimulus. Massaging skin causes a feeling of firm pressure, and scratching or lightly pricking of skin corresponding mild sensations. All of these stimuli, when correctly applied, are followed, after their cessation, by a heavy, numb, aching or burning feeling. These occur in the part stimulated, and may also radiate some distance to adjacent areas or across the midline of the body.

Insertion of an acupuncture needle is nearly painfree. There may be a slight prick as the point passes through the skin, but once this stage is over the patient frequently does not know the needle is in situ. It is very much less painful than having a conventional hypodermic injection. This is because the hypodermic needle has a cutting edge at the point whereas the acupuncture needle is rounded at the end or, as the medical jargon has it, 'atraumatic'. For this reason there is almost never any bleeding associated with piqure. Once again, after the needle has been in position for a while in an acupuncture point, and particularly if it has been manipulated or stimulated electrically, a feeling of heavy numbness occurs which the Chinese call t'chi. There is considerable evidence that unless this feeling occurs the acupuncture stimulus will not be so successful, and so the acupuncturist will often question his patient on this point and may continue to manipulate the needle until t'chi is experienced.

After the needle is removed and the area massaged with a little alcohol to cleanse it and discourage bleeding, the warm heavy feeling will persist, sometimes for several hours. If the patient inspects his skin at the site of acupuncture stimulation, whether by needle, cautery or massage, there will be seen to be a red flare at this point due to dilatation of the minute blood vessels running in the skin. There may also be, right at the centre of the red region, a tiny raised weal which marks the actual site of needle insertion or other stimulation. These phenomena are quite natural, indeed necessary, effects of the treatment. Again, they will last for minutes to hours afterwards, the flare sometimes persisting into the following day.

With the greatest of care it is sometimes impossible to avoid nicking one of the tiny veins that run in the skin. If this occurs, a small bruise may form, with perhaps a swelling, and this will last as long as any bruise caused by accidental injury.

One special case needs to be mentioned as giving rise to sensations which are different from the rest. If electrical stimulation of the needles is used a tingling feeling is caused, like any mild electric shock. The acupuncturist can alter the intensity of this by regulating the current and waveform of the output of the equipment he uses to stimulate the points. It is common practice for the stimulus intensity gradually to be increased until it just starts to be painful, and then turned down again slightly. There is no point in being a martyr in this situation, and the patient should indicate as soon as pain is felt.

Once again I must stress that acupuncture is not painful. Indeed, it is well known by practitioners that a painful stimulus is much less effective than a painless one; and there are good neurophysiological reasons for this.

Could My Problem Get Worse?

There is a famous saying which applies to very many aspects of medicine: 'there is no always or never in medicine'. Wise medical students actually use this axiom in answering multiple choice examination questions. When the question is phrased as say 'myocardial infarction is always associated with T wave inversion in lead II of the electrocardiagram — true or false?' a student really need know nothing about heart disease or ECG's to realize that the correct answer is 'false'. T wave inversions often occur; but not always. In medicine nearly anything is possible and the true science and art of the subject is learning, with experience, to balance all of the possibilities and arrive at the most likely diagnosis, probably the best treatment, the most frequent prognosis and so on.

The reason for this lengthy preamble is that I want the reader to appreciate that whilst the worsening of symptoms is unlikely to occur, to any important extent and for anything more than a short period, this cannot completely be ruled out as impossible. Actually a temporary worsening of the symptoms is a fairly common occurrence after the first treatment. It seems to come on fairly rapidly, and lasts a few hours to a few days and, when it does occur, it is usually a sign that the outcome will eventually be beneficial. It may be interpreted as a sign that the treatment has affected points which are linked in some way with the illness to be cured, whereas if the acupuncturist had inadvertently chosen points which had not associated at all with the illness, there is likely to be no effect whatsoever.

Many acupuncturists feel that patients who show this kind of response may be classified as 'strong reactors' to acupuncture stimulation and that this is an indication to use a very mild treatment. As with many drugs the optimal doses vary, so with acupuncture some people need stronger or weaker treatments. Just because a teaspoonful is good for you, it does not mean a bucketful would be better! A substantial proportion, say 10 per cent to 15 per cent, of patients treated with acupuncture respond abnormally strongly to even a mild treatment. (Another 10 per cent to 15 per cent respond very little to even the most vigorous manipulations.)

This probably just represents one tail of the normal distribution curve in the population of response to treatment; but it does mean that the strength of the treatment has to be gauged according to the individual patient's needs. Patients who will probably require only a gentle treatment are often fit young men, particularly athletic types, those with a high intelligence, sensitive and artistic individuals, and those who have a history of allergy to various things. These patients often feel faint during the actual treatment, and the wise practitioner makes sure they are lying down before using the needles, whereby fainting is avoided. Very young patients are also rather hypersensitive; whereas old people require a stronger stimulation. Lastly, patients who are debilitated by their illness will often only tolerate a mild stimulus on the first few occasions. When their condition improves, the stimulus intensity can be increased. All in all it is better to give too weak a stimulus than too strong a one, especially during the first treatment, since the intensity can always be increased later. In any case, in treating acupuncture points we are trying to press the right buttons, not smash the control panel!

As explained, too strong a stimulus is sometimes one of the factors predisposing to a temporary reactive increase of the symptoms. This sort of reaction is much rarer following treatments after the first; although one of my patients, who happened to be a doctor himself, found during a course of treatment that the sessions which helped him most always gave rise to a brief deterioration of his backache before the eventual improvement. Needling lower body points is less likely to cause a reaction of this kind than treating those above the waist, and the reaction very rarely occurs after auriculotherapy.

Still, what patients and doctors alike fear is a permanent

worsening of some illness as a result of acupuncture treatment, and this fortunately seems to be extremely rare, if not unknown.

Another rather rare occurence is for some new symptom to arise during the course of treatment, although it is often very difficult to decide whether this is due to progression or change in the illness or to treatment itself. For instance, in the treatment of nasosinusitis it is not unknown for the nasal discharge to be more profuse for a while although the pain and stuffiness which characterize this condition may be much reduced. Once again, when this happens, it usually signifies the outcome will eventually be satisfactory, and is an adjunct to the healing process. Nevertheless, all such incidents should, of course, be reported to the doctor.

Could I Become Addicted to Acupuncture?

This question often seems to arise in the minds of patients, although it may not be phrased in precisely the same way. What is usually meant is, given that the outcome of treatment in any particular case is extremely hard to predict, and that fairly long courses may be necessary to produce or maintain benefit, is there a chance that there will be a need for regular treatment for the rest of life? This would have obvious implications in terms of cost and inconvenience. The fact is, that very nearly all patients require the pattern of treatment previously referred to: a short burst of frequent treatment followed by top up ones at long intervals, which quite rapidly lengthen further. Finally no more treatment is required.

Once a condition disappears under treatment, it is unlikely to recur after treatment has stopped. If it is reduced in severity, it probably will not get worse again. Of course, the whole cycle of treatment, from induction to maintenance, may take a year or longer to accomplish, but it seems exceedingly rare for treatment to continue to be necessary for ever after, let alone for treatment to be required increasingly often, or with increasing intensity, to maintain an improvement. In any case, where this did happen, it would be regarded by the acupuncturist as an indication that the case was not suitable for this form of therapy, and the patient would be referred back to his own doctor for alternative possibilities to be explored.

There is a grey borderline area in which treatment to control an illness is required a little too often, or too long, for it to be sensible or convenient for a patient to attend the surgery for its administration. It is under these circumstances that the practitioner will consider instructing the patient in self-therapy by massage, a plum blossom needle or electrical stimulation.

What Are the Dangers?

All medical treatments have the potential for causing harm as well as benefit. Doctors (and patients) must carefully evaluate the 'risk/benefit ratio' in deciding whether to go ahead. Some severe surgical operations have an extremely high ratio. Perhaps 50 per cent of patients undergoing some major operation may not be helped and may even die. The operation will be justified if it is the *only* way of treating a life-threatening disease. An example of such a procedure would be heart transplantation in a patient with a very short life expectancy due to their cardiac disease.

Acupuncture, as stated already, is fortunately a very safe procedure in skilled hands. Nevertheless, there are some hazards which are possible, and these fall into three principal categories: the chance of introducing infection, the risk of damaging bodily structures, and the risk of masking underlying disease by abolishing its symptoms.

Infection

The surface of the body, the skin, may be thought of as the body's first line of defence against infection by micro-organisms. There are many viruses and bacteria which can cause harm once inside the body; but they must first find a portal of entry. They can be ingested with food or water, or inhaled, but in these cases they meet at once specialized bodily secretions and cells whose function is to deal with such intruders. For instance, in the lungs there are so-called 'phagocytic' cells, which engulf and destroy micro-organisms, and in the stomach the highly acidic gastric secretions kill microbes. When the skin is breached and organisms are introduced directly into the tissues underneath, and thence into the bloodstream, there is a greater risk of the infection taking hold and causing an illness. Even in this situation there are many bodily mechanisms for repelling the attack including, as elsewhere, phagocytic cells and special chemicals. Still, the risk is intrinsically higher, and when an acupuncture needle is pushed through the skin, as in any surgical procedure, scrupulous cleanliness is essential.

The first stage in this is the sterilization of the needle itself. Boiling is not sufficient since some organisms, particularly those causing hepatitis, are not destroyed by this means. Sterilization with steam in an autoclave or with hot air or radiation is essential. Some acupuncturists use disposable needles, which are thrown away after one use.

The patient's skin is sterilized with an alcohol swab, although there is actually some evidence to show that this is not so important as was hitherto believed. Actual pre-existing skin infections, such as impetigo, boils or carbuncles, are a contra-indication to acupuncture treatment at the site affected. With adequate precautions such as these, the introduction of infection by acupuncture treatment is not a problem.

Damage to Body Structures

The possibility of causing injury by inadvertently needling structures under the skin is a much greater hazard and demands a full knowledge of anatomy on the part of the practitioner. Nerves and blood vessels (particularly arteries) are amongst the most vulnerable structures, although other organs such as the lung, are also at risk. There has been a number of cases of pneumothorax reported in the medical literature due to improper placing of acupuncture needles at the top of the front of the chest, where the lungs come very close to the surface. In this condition, air escapes from a punctured lung into the sac which surrounds it. Pressure builds up and can eventually collapse the lung, causing asphyxia.

If nerves are damaged by needling or other treatments, the

end result can be very unpleasant. Neuralgic pains, with muscle wasting or loss of sensation can occur in the part the nerve supplies.

These kinds of hazards can be avoided easily if the position of subcutaneous structures is known. Obviously, some areas of the body are more critical than others in this respect. The best guarantee of safety in this matter is to consult a medically qualified acupuncturist, who has received the normal extensive training in human anatomy which forms part of the medical school syllabus.

The Risk of Masking Underlying Disease

Acupuncture provides the means to reduce or abolish pain, stiffness, muscle spasm and many other unpleasant effects which are caused by human illness. In some instances signs and symptoms of the illness go because the illness itself is cured. In others, the underlying pathological process is only partly modified, or unchanged. This leads to the possibility that a patient may be unaware that his illness is continuing to progress, perhaps with very serious consequences, because the symptoms have been suppressed. For instance, if a person with backache is treated by acupuncture and obtains relief, in over ninety per cent of instances this can only be a good thing. By far the largest proportion of backache is caused by essentially self-limiting disorders such as a prolapsed intervertebral disc, a muscle strain or the spraining of a ligament. However, a rare cause of backache is a tumour of the bones of the spine, and if the pain from this is suppressed, this may delay the patient from taking steps to obtain effective treatment to prevent tumour growth and spread.

Of course, this situation is not unique to acupuncture. It applies to all forms of effective treatment which provides symptomatic relief, including osteopathy, physiotherapy, treatment with drugs, and so on. It is absolutely essential for the acupuncture practitioner to think of the underlying diagnosis, and not just treat the symptoms alone, and this is something which the medically trained practitioner would regard as second nature.

What If I Do Not Think the Treatment is Working?

Acupuncture is not a panacea or 'cure all'. It is not worth trying for some illnesses; in others the chances of success are small; and in still others, which normally respond excellently, there will be occasional inexplicable failures. The acupuncturist will keep close tabs on progress of the treatment, making adjustments when required, or even abandoning the method if it is clearly failing. But in many cases he will rely heavily on his patient's account of the effects of each treatment. Headache is an entirely subjective phenomenon which cannot be measured by the medical recording equipment which exists today, so it is necessary for the patient to describe to his doctor, at each consultation, the response of this symptom to the treatment previously given. Then the doctor will maintain or alter the treatment accordingly. There is a very natural inclination in many patients to 'help the doctor' by scouring the memory for any signs of an improvement, and by playing down things which might suggest that matters are stable or even getting worse. After all there is, or should be, a good personal relationship between them. The patient will not wish to disappoint the doctor, and may even be a little in awe of him and afraid of incurring displeasure. On the other hand, the patient is also extremely anxious himself to improve; so it is very easy for the picture to become distorted.

In an earlier chapter I described the double blind clinical trial which compares two or more treatments to see which is best. In this, neither doctor nor patient knows which treatment the patient is getting, so there is no possibility of this kind of bias creeping in. This is clearly not possible in the normal therapeutic situation. For these reasons it is vitally important for the patient to be as honest as he can with the acupuncturist. If he does not feel the treatment is helping he should say so at once, so something new can be tried. Of course, instant miracles should not be expected, and a sufficient time for a fair trial of the treatment has to be allowed.

How Do I Pay?

The labourer is worthy of his hire. Doctors accept patients for treatment, and in return are paid a fee for their professional services. The fee may be paid by the government, by the National Health Service; by a medical insurance organization, such as the British United Provident Association, or the Private Patients Plan; or by the patient himself.

An intending patient may find an acupuncturist operating within the NHS, either in general practice or in hospital medicine. (These are rare, for various reasons, some of which have been alluded to previously.) If this is the case no fee will be payable to the doctor, who seeks his remuneration from the Health Service which employs him. This point should be made clear before or during the first consultation; and if the patient is not sure of the situation, he should certainly ask.

The alternative case concerns the doctor who operates privately, as an independent contractor, just like a barrister, accountant or architect. In this case he will expect the patient to pay for his services, either directly or through his membership of an insurance company. The practitioner's scale of fees should be determined at the outset; and there is no need to feel shy about asking the practitioner's receptionist or the practitioner himself about it. It is worth asking, at the same time, whether payment at each consultation is preferred or whether an account will be submitted at intervals or at the end of the course of treatment. Some patients themselves prefer one or other method of payment and there will normally be no reason why their wishes cannot be accommodated.

Where an insurance organization is involved, the company will wish the patient to send the account which the doctor has submitted for payment, as well as a form completed by doctor and patient, detailing the medical condition and form of treatment carried out. The patient pays the doctor and is then reimbursed by the insurance company, usually very quickly. It is important to note that various companies practices vary somewhat as to whom they consider as specialist medical practitioners within the meaning of their rules governing reimbursement of fees. The criterion often seems to be whether or not the practitioner has an appointment in hospital, although he may have seen the patient in his private rooms at home or elsewhere. Of course, only medically qualified practitioners are considered. The only safe course of action, if there is any doubt as to whether an acupuncturist's fees can be reclaimed, is to contact the organization, explain the situation and ask for a ruling.

Chapter 6

How Did Acupuncture Originate?

Quite where and when acupuncture started is not known. The earliest book on the subject dates to the time of the Yellow Emperor Huang Ti, who lived in the Warring States period in China, 475 to 221 BC. The book was prepared for him, and is called the *Nei Ching* or *Classic of Internal Medicine*. In it he gives instructions to his physicians, as follows: 'Huang Ti speaks to Ch'i Po: I, who am chief of a great people and who should receive taxes from them, find myself afflicted by not being able to collect them because my people are sick. I desire, therefore, that the employment of remedies cease and that only the needles be used. I order that this matter be transmitted to all future generations and that the laws concerning it be clearly defined, so that it will be easy to practice it, hard to forget it, and that it will not be abandoned in the future. Besides this, the actual modalities are to be accurately observed so that the way to research will be opened.'

Early copies of the book are still in existence, and it has been reprinted in modern times as the *Yellow Emperor's Classic of Internal Medicine*.

Another book which records primitive stone instruments for acupuncture is *The Book of Mountains and Seas,* the *Shan Hai Jing,* written more than 2,000 years ago. Part of this reads: 'In the Kaoshih mountains are rich deposits . . . of stone suitable for making needles.'

The Chinese clearly became aware of acupuncture a very considerable time ago. The story of how this occurred may well be apocryphal, but is an interesting one. It is said that a soldier was pierced by an arrow in battle. He survived his injury and, on recovery, a long-standing illness had disappeared. Observation and experiment leading from this incident caused the development of the whole system of medical treatment we know as acupuncture. It was noticed that certain organs were associated with specific points on the skin which often became tender when the organs were diseased and which could be used for the treatment of these disorders. The points appeared to be linked by imaginary lines which could be drawn on the skin: the meridians or 'ching'. The linkage between diseases, acupuncture points and channels was explained by a complex philosophical system invoking disorders of energy disturbance within the body, which could be diagnosed in various ways, such as examination of the skin, of the tongue and of the twelve radial pulses. The points and meridians were actually thought of as channelling energy called ch'i (broadly, of a positive yang or a negative ying kind) from one part of the body to the other. The flow of energy could be regulated by inserting needles in the appropriate points, and by other manipulations. It was considered that the body was endowed with a certain quantity of energy at birth which was depleted by the activities involved in daily living. However, it could be restored by eating and drinking. Disturbances of energy circulation cause disease and, of course, an absence of it, death.

Development of Acupuncture Needles

The history of acupuncture in China is really the history of the needles of various materials which were utilized, since these artefacts can be used to date the practice and locate it geographically. Instruments for puncturing the skin made of splinters of sharp stone have been found in sites from the neolithic period. Later other materials were used, such as pottery, bone and wood. When craftsmanship in metal developed, needles were made which were not unlike those used today (see Figure 7). In the Shang dynasty, from 1558 BC, bronze was used for a variety of fine articles, and metal needles gradually replaced the porcelain ones. Later iron, gold and silver needles developed.

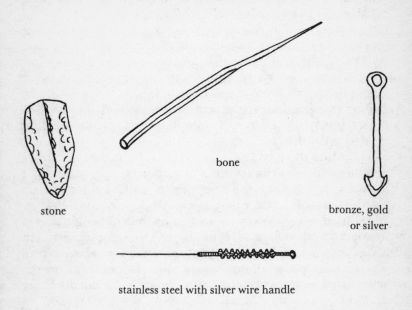

stone

bone

bronze, gold or silver

stainless steel with silver wire handle

Figure 7. Development of acupuncture needles.

Chinese works through the centuries record the use of acupuncture by various physicians for treating the rich and famous. In *Shi Ji* (historical records) there is an account of a physician Pien Cheuh, living several hundred years before Christ, using acupuncture to cure a comatose patient. This doctor wrote the *Nan Ching* (difficult classic) which expanded the earlier *nei Ching*. Between AD 250 and 600 acupuncture developed rapidly in China, and further books and even coloured charts describing the channels and points for the treatment of various conditions appeared. A notable advance in the Tang dynasty (AD 618 to 907) was the discovery that tender areas of skin, called the ah shi points, could be used for acupuncture treatment, supplementing the acupuncture points traditionally described. In the Sung, Kin and Yuan periods (AD 960 to 1368) further important treatises were written, and the acupuncture points were listed and categorized. A total of 657 classical points was recorded and the Emperor Wei Te Wang ordered the casting of two life size bronze figures, the T'ong Jen, which illustrated the precise courses of the meridians and locations of the points. The statues were used for teaching, and smaller copies in other materials are employed to this date in training acupuncturists. During examinations the practitioner must find acupuncture points unerringly by blindly needling holes in the models, through a covering of rice paper!

The Ming dynasty (1368 to 1644) was a period of further development of acupuncture, but, during the years that followed, it was extensively suppressed in China for various political reasons. The rulers of the Ching dynasty (1644 to 1911) tried to ban treatment by this method although, due to its widespread popular acceptance, they were not successful in abolishing its use. It was during this period that acupuncture was first introduced into Europe, first in Germany in the seventeenth century and then into France in the middle of the nineteenth century. Much of the early dissemination of knowledge of acupuncture was by Jesuit missionaries returning from China in the 1700s. The Chinese government again banned traditional medicine in 1929, but once more failed to suppress it completely.

Moxibustion

The variant of acupuncture called moxibustion probably has a much shorter history. Its origins are obscure but it was first recorded in China in the northern Sung dynasty (AD 960) and it was further categorized and defined early in the eleventh century. Actually, the word moxibustion derives from the Japanese word mokusa meaning burning herb, and the early Chinese refer to these techniques as cauterizations. Around the same time anatomical dissections started to be practised in China and a careful search for the imaginary entities known as the meridians began, and continues to this day.

Acupuncture in Modern China

Since the second World War there has been a considerable redevelopment of acupuncture and moxibustion in China, with an appreciation of their complementary role to modern methods. Fittingly, the Chinese were amongst the first to institute proper programmes of scientific research into its mode of action. In China a great impetus to the development of acupuncture has been the relative poverty of the country and the lack of conventionally trained physicians, of drugs and of medical equipment. The medical care of many of the more rural areas has depended extensively on medical auxiliaries with a slight basic training in hygiene, medical and surgical treatment, herbal medicine and acupuncture. These 'barefoot doctors' live in and travel around communes, advising and treating the farm workers.

Development of acupuncture and other traditional Chinese medical arts was one of Mao Tse-Tung's aims, particularly following the experience of his army during the so-called 'Long March' of 1934-5, during which such techniques played an important role in maintaining the troops health and freedom from epidemics. Today acupuncture is still used widely by the general population, and needles and other equipment for acupuncture and moxibustion can be purchased in shops as readily as say aspirin for a headache in the West. The popular view of the efficacy of the method can be judged from the proverb 'a single needle can free the body from 10,000 maladies'.

Japan

In Japan, Chinese medical techniques were practised extensively from about AD 1600 but, in an attempt to encourage development of more modern ideas, they were banned in the late nineteenth century. (In 1884 Western medical departments were instituted in many Japanese universities.) But suppression of acupuncture was not at all successful, as in China, because of the value placed on it by the general population in the treatment of commonplace disorders as well as serious disease. Today a much more balanced approach pertains, with both traditional and modern techniques practised and studied, often side by side.

The Spread to the West

One of the most important factors in the promulgation of knowledge of acupuncture in the West in modern times was the activities of the French diplomat, Soulie de Morant. De Morant was a great lover of things Chinese and wrote many works on acupuncture in the 1940s. As a result, the technique was brought to the attention of physicians in many countries, including France, USSR, Britain, Italy, Germany and Argentina.

A more recent influence was the upsurge of interest in Chinese matters which occurred at the time of President Nixon and 'Ping Pong Diplomacy'. In 1971 a famous American commentator James Reston, visiting Peking with his wife, suddenly contracted acute appendicitis. He required emergency surgery, which was expertly carried out under conventional local analgesia. Two days later, when he suffered post operative abdominal pain, he was treated by acupuncture. Needling of points near the knees and elbows was combined with moxibustion. Much to the surprise and interest of Mr Reston and his wife, the result was relief of the pain. He wrote later: 'I have seen the past, and it works'. The Restons travelled to various parts of China and visited hospitals and communes in which acupuncture was used for the treatment of infantile poliomyelitis and tuberculosis, dental procedures such as tooth extractions, and major chest surgery such as the removal of a lung. On their return, their description of what they had witnessed caused a considerable stir and did much to focus public and professional attention on acupuncture.

As a result of the growth of knowledge about acupuncture in western countries numbers of professional associations and study groups have been formed and programmes for research into the subject have been commenced. This is particularly the case in the Far East, in Japan and China and also in the USSR, the USA and, latterly and to a smaller extent, in the United Kingdom.

Chapter 7

How Does Acupuncture Work?

This question is easily answered. We do not know! However, there are many examples of effective medical treatments which act by mechanisms as yet unknown; and this does not detract from their usefulness. In fact, with acupuncture, the situation is not quite as mysterious as all that. There is an accumulating weight of evidence derived from careful scientific research that is beginning to clarify the underlying changes which needling the skin produces. I shall try to explain some of the evidence as simply as possible, but an understanding of this is not necessary for a patient to benefit from treatment, or even for a doctor to administer it. Both can simply accept acupuncture at face value as a form of therapy which, used skilfully in suitable cases, is capable of producing considerable benefit.

Suggestion? Hypnosis? Charlatanism?
It was at first suggested that acupuncture represented a rather complicated way of producing results by suggestion or hypnosis. As discussed in an earlier chapter, many patients will show considerable improvement even when treated with a quite inactive substance or technique (the placebo response). This is particularly the case if the treatment is accompanied by strong reassurance and predictions of success by the doctor. However, certain classes of patients are not at all

susceptible to this effect, and the fact that acupuncture works in them prevents this from explaining its efficacy. This is not to say that suggestibility does not play a part in the response of a patient to acupuncture, as with any medical treatment, but it cannot nearly be the whole story. Babies and very young children, as well as animals, do not know they are expected to get better when they are treated medically. Indeed they do not even know they are being treated. Acupuncture works well in many paediatric and veterinary conditions, so we must seek some alternative mechanism to hypnosis or suggestion.

In general, alterations to the body's physiological state can be caused chemically or electrically. (In fact the distinction is very blurred, because electrical changes have at their roots changes in the chemistry of the nerve cells which conduct electricity.)

When an influence on the body is mediated chemically it has certain characteristics, especially a rather slow onset of action. Acupuncture often works very quickly indeed, and so scientists have looked to other ways in which the body's functions can be altered: by electrical changes occurring in the nervous system. Classical oriental acupuncturists have, for many hundreds of years, explained acupuncture as invoking energy changes in a system of conducting pathways: the acupuncture meridians. These were supposed to be channels linking points associated with given organ systems in the body. Intercommunications were said to exist between the various channels, and the whole system formed a network of great complexity. Anatomists and microscopists have searched carefully for these minute channels, but without success.

A Korean, Kim Bon Hang claimed to have found ducts and corpuscles forming the acupuncture meridians, but careful investigation showed that he had only rediscovered channels well known to exist and to have other functions: the lymphatics. It is exceedingly unlikely that generations of scientists have overlooked some system of communicating pathways other than the lymphatics, blood vessels and nerves, and we must rely on these known structures to account for the way acupuncture stimuli can affect the body.

The Nervous System

As stated the speed of response suggests nervous mediation. It is very well known that the state of functioning of internal organs can affect the skin. For instance inflammation of organs in the abdomen can give rise to pain felt in the skin, areas tender to the touch, and even muscle spasm, even some distance from the diseased structure. The blood vessels in the skin can also be affected and become dilated or constricted. These effects are caused through nervous pathways called, logically enough, viscero-cutaneous reflexes. The word reflex implies that the changes are not under conscious control; although a person may be aware that they are happening. It is thought to be in this way that the so called 'trigger points' so important in acupuncture are caused. Pain felt at some site away from where the pathological change is actually occurring is called 'referred pain'. Reference of pain can occur from an internal organ to the skin. It can also occur from muscles or joints to the skin, or from one patch of skin to another.

The nerve supply of the skin, muscles, joints, and organs in the chest or abdomen arises at different levels in the central core of nervous tissue which runs up the backbone, called the spinal cord. Nerve roots pass through the bones of the spine and form divisions which get progressively finer and finer as they approach the tissues. Impulses taking sensations centrally towards the spinal cord and brain pass from the tissues. 'Motor' impulses are transmitted in the opposite direction, and form the instructions which cause glands to secrete, muscles to contract and blood vessels to change diameter. In referral of pain, transmission usually occurs to a place which lies within the area supplied by nerves arising from the same part of the spinal cord as the primary site of disease. However, reference to remote areas, even on the other side of the body, can occur. It is probable that reference is caused by relay cells in the spinal cord or brain being shared by fibres arising both from the primary site and the site at which the referred pain is felt. The central mechanisms which allow us to experience the sensation of pain interpret the pain as coming from the normal area and not the diseased part, as in fact is the case. Pain referred to the secondary site in this way sometimes causes local release of chemicals which inflame nerve endings at the site of reference. This then makes them pass secondary pain messages of their own and so reinforces the whole effect.

Counter-Irritation

Pathways running in the opposite direction also exist: the cutaneo-visceral reflexes. By involving these, stimulation of the skin in various ways can affect the functioning of the internal viscera. For instance, irritation of the skin of the ear canal can cause slowing of the heart, and even collapse. Effects on the blood flow and motility of the intestine can be caused similarly. It is presumably in this way that acupuncture stimulation affects the functioning of the viscera and alters the body's responses to its environment.

Additionally, anaesthetizing, heating, cooling or mildly injuring areas of skin will often abolish pain arising from other sites. It is common knowledge that cold sprays will ease many muscular pains, and infra-red lamps and other forms of heating are also effective. Certain forms of 'counter-irritation' are as old as medicine itself. In these, a strong stimulus, perhaps even a painful one, is applied to the skin either close to the site of the pain or at some other position. When this is applied, the original pain is eased, and this reduction of pain may persist for long periods afterwards. For many hundreds of years in Britain, beating the lower back with prickly branches has been used as a treatment for backache. Nettles have also been used. Cynics would say that this is so painful that it just takes one's mind off the backache, but that this cannot be the whole story is shown by the persistence of relief after the counter-irritation has ceased. Another example of counter-irritation used through the ages to modern times is simply rubbing a part after it has been injured. Everyday experience shows that this is a very effective way of relieving pain. Western and oriental massage also acts in the same way when used to relieve painful conditions; and many massage techniques are very close indeed to acupuncture, stimulating areas of skin rich in acupuncture points!

Various theories have been suggested to account for the phenomenon of counter-irritation, mainly involving a form of competitive inhibition at nervous relays in the spinal cord and brain. Let me explain. In the same way that sharing of a linking nerve cell by fibres arising from two different sites can lead to referral of pain from a diseased area to a patch of normal skin, shared neurones can allow pain relief. If stimulating an area of skin could affect the linking nerve cell to render it less able to pass pain impulses from the site of disease, the sensation of pain which occurs within the brain would be reduced. This is just what is thought to happen. The skin sites which, when stimulated, give rise to the best responses are of course acupuncture points.

For a long time the way in which the linking nerve cells were rendered incapable of passing pain messages was thought of as 'overloading'. It was presumed that they were so bombarded with messages from skin stimulation that they were saturated and could not deal with the pain impulses arising elsewhere. This is the case; but it is not the whole story. There has now been a considerable amount of research on how this happens, which is of great interest and importance in other branches of medicine. Firstly, it might be thought that a stimulus strong enough to saturate relay capacity in this way would be, in itself, excruciatingly painful. Two possible explanations for this have been suggested. The peripheral stimulus might affect not pain receptors and nerves, but those of some other sense. The nerve endings which subserve sensation of joint position, 'proprioceptors', have been suggested. But proprioceptors are not found outside muscles, joints and tendons, and it would seem that only pain endings are sufficiently ubiquitous to be implicated.

The 'Gate Control' Theory

The second theory, which was first proposed in 1965, postulates a 'gate control mechanism' at the level of the linking nerve cells (See Figure 8). Electrophysiological experiments show that the nerve fibres associated with pain are mostly fine and conduct impulses slowly, but that some large, rapidly conducting fibres are also involved. It is probable that acupuncture stimulation predominantly causes large fibre activity which is not sensed as painful but which 'shuts the

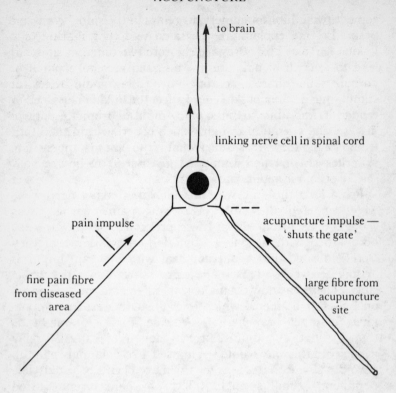

Figure 8. Gate control theory.

gate'. That is it prevents the linking nerve cell passing true
pain sensations which arise from the site of disease and are
normally transmitted by slower moving impulses passing in
fine nerve fibres. In other words stimulation of the skin so as to
fire the fast conducting pain fibres would impede pain
impulses from passing centrally from an area which shares the
same relays.

However, too strong a skin stimulus would start to involve
the small fibres arising from this site. When there is an
increase in the ratio of small to large fibre traffic the 'gate' is
opened and pain is felt. The excessive skin stimulus itself is felt
to be painful but, more important, the relay is allowed to pass
pain from the diseased area too. This theory accords well with

clinical practice in acupuncture in which, as I have said before, a very strong stimulus is often not nearly as effective as a weaker one. Once pain is felt the treatment can often make things worse. If the stimulus causes pain then presumably the resulting small fibre valley facilitates transmission across the relay instead of impeding it.

As was stated earlier, the electrical activity of the nervous system has chemical changes at its foundation. It has long been known that at the endings of nerves, where they join to other nerves or to organs which carry out their instructions, the electrical impulse jumps the gap by means of a chemical form of transmission. Minute quantities of various substances are released which excite the next nerve in line, or the effector organ. There are many such 'neuro-transmitter substances', for example non-adrenaline and acetyl-choline. Quite recently a whole new class has been discovered, which seems to modulate the responses of nerve cells to the classical neuro-transmitters and to be heavily involved in the transmission of pain information. These are the so called 'endogenous opioids'.

Endogenous Opioids

The class of powerful pain killers used in medicine known as the opiates includes heroine, morphine and pethidine. They are able to relieve severe pain, but for many years after their discovery little was known about their mode of action. It is usually true to say that when a drug exerts its effecs it must first bind on to receptor sites on the cells of the tissue where the effect will occur. The opiate analgesics are no exception and it was felt highly unlikely that the good Lord had provided us with opiate receptor sites in the nervous system simply in case one day we discovered these drugs and started to use them therapeutically. In other words the fact that such sites occur is strong evidence that they are there for another reason: the binding of some similar chemical substances which do occur naturally within the body.

A few years ago these endogenous naturally occurring opiates were discovered; the endopioids. Many slightly different varieties have since been found, and they are now sub-divided into larger molecules, the endorphins, and smaller ones, the enkephalins. Both consist of chains made up of amino acids, the building blocks of proteins. Discovery of these substances has provided us with an explanation of many of the interesting phenomena of medicine as well as an opportunity for various forms of new drug therapy. For instance the symptoms suffered by heroin addicts when their drug is withdrawn are explained. The large quantities of exogenous opiates taken by the addict supress the production of the endogenous naturally occurring forms in their nervous systems. When their addiction is under treatment the drug is withdrawn. The mechanisms which produce endopioids cannot prevent a considerable drop in the levels present when heroin was being taken, and various unpleasant symptoms result, such as sweating, hallucinations, intense anxiety and abdominal cramps.

'Neuromodulators' are produced very quickly in tiny amounts which are then promptly reabsorbed or broken down so that they do not go on acting. In this respect they are quite different from the other chemicals which modify bodily functions: the hormones secreted by 'ductless glands' such as the thyroid and adrenal. These are produced slowly and for long periods, and are carried around the bloodstream exerting their action for hours or even days.

We may now examine some of the evidence which supports the theories outlined above. Firstly, if local analgesic solution (like that used by the dentist) is injected into the base of an acupuncture point before it is needled, the treatment is ineffective. The same applies to treatments carried out in areas which lack sensation because of a stroke, or in areas where the nerve supply has been disrupted by radiotherapy, scarring, a viral infection or a surgical procedure. Thus, an intact nerve supply, running from the skin to the spinal cord, is essential for acupuncture to work, and it is clear that the stimulus sets up afferent nervous impulses which run in the pain pathways from the periphery towards the central nervous system, and, ultimately, the brain.

These impulses pass through an area at the back of the spinal cord called the 'dorsal horn'. By special biochemical techniques linked with microscopic examination, it can be shown that the nerve cells here secrete enkephalins; one of the two classes of endogenous opiates previously referred to. Other such endopioid secreting cells can be found in various higher portions of the central nervous system, and they lie along the pathways associated with the transmission of pain sensation. From the dorsal horn, nerve fibres cross the midline and pass through lateral tracts running from the spine to the region of the base of the brain called the thalamus. Diseases of this region may give rise to a particularly unpleasant kind of pain, which is extremely hard to treat. Outflow from the thalamus passes to the cerebral cortex, in which the sensation of pain is felt. Endopioid secreting cells are found in the thalamus and the cortex, and also in the 'limbic system' which is involved in the emotional response to pain.

It is almost certainly secretion of endogenous opiates which close the 'gate' previously referred to, inhibiting the onward transmission of pain impulses in many parts of the pathways from peripheral nerve endings to the cerebral cortex. One piece of evidence which shows this was discovered in China in 1974. The nerve cells in the spinal cord and brain are bathed in a nutrient medium called the cerebro-spinal fluid. It is possible to show, by experiments in rabbits, that the pain of nipping the skin of the foot with a pair of tweezers can be inhibited by acupuncture stimulation, using a needle inserted at the appropriate site.

An interesting feature of these experiments is that excessive acupuncture stimulation, far from reducing the pain caused by pinching the skin, actually seems to make it worse. Additionally, if the rabbit is agitated, perhaps because its usual handler is replaced by a stranger, acupuncture stimulation is less effective. If some of the cerebro-spinal fluid of a rabbit treated by acpuncture is infused around the spinal cord of another rabbit having a similar painful stimulus, but not receiving acupuncture, it too is protected from feeling pain. The clear conclusion to be drawn is that the cerebro-spinal fluid of the acupuncture-treated rabbit is modified in some way so that it can suppress pain impulse transmission in the spinal cord of an untreated animal.

Further studies in humans since carried out in the West have shown that the modification consists of endopioid secretion, and that the endopioid containing fluid acts as a natural analgesic or pain killer. Identification and measurement of the various endogenous opioids are technically very difficult, and considerable caution needs to be exercised in interpreting data in the medical literature. However, in a number of studies, acupuncture stimulation has been found to be followed by increases in the concentration of endopioids in the cerebrospinal fluid. What is more, by tapping off fluid at different levels, the secretion of endopioids can be shown to occur only at the level of the spinal cord involved in the particular acupuncture stimulation given. Thus, stimulation of points on the lower limbs causes endopioid secretion from the lower lumbar parts of the spinal cord which can be detected in fluid collected from this area; whereas stimulation of points on the upper limbs would increase the endopioid concentration only of cerebro-spinal fluid collected from the region of the neck.

Pathways running downwards from the cerebral cortex to the spinal cord also exist. Again, endopioid secretion along the route of this diminishes pain transmission, and this may well be the mechanism which explains the soldier injured in battle, or the footballer on the soccer pitch, who does not feel his pain in the heat of the moment but collapses once the battle or match is over. Under these circumstances, the cerebral cortex sends down impulses which dull the pain of injury; and this mechanism has obvious value in enabling a seriously injured person to remain active and mobile when he must, in the 'fight or flight' situation. Similar descending pathways may account for the great muscular strength which people can manifest under extremely stressful circumstances, as in the case of the mother who was able to lift clear a car which was crushing her child.

Opiate Antagonists

Not only are there drugs which occupy opiate receptors to cause their therapeutic effect, there are also 'opiate antagonists' which bind to the same receptors but are therapeutically inactive. Drug receptor theory is often explained using the analogy of a lock and its key. Effective drugs are like keys which occupy the lock and can turn it. Antagonists occupy the lock, but they do not turn it. What is more, they block it, preventing another key, which will turn the lock, from being inserted. One effective opiate antagonist is the drug naloxone. When this is administered it occupies spinal receptors to endopioids and competes with them at these sites. It will come as no surprise to learn that many of the effects of acupuncture, mediated by endopioid secretion, are reversed by simultaneous administration of naloxone. This 'naloxone reversibility' is, in itself, strong evidence that endopioid secretion occurs following acupuncture stimulation.

Direct electrical stimulation of various places in the ascending pain pathways can be carried out by inserting fine wire electrodes into these areas, in experimental animals or in human patients. Such stimulation of the dorsal columns of the spinal cord or of the grey matter in the brain stem can be used clinically to relieve severe chronic pain. Once again it can be shown that stimulation causes release of endopioids; and the pain relief is partially reversible by naloxone. Because of the difficulties and hazards of inserting electrodes into the spinal cord and the brain it has been attempted to obtain similar results from electrodes applied to the surface of the skin in various positions (transcutaneous electrical nerve stimulation: TENS). It is becoming increasingly obvious that both this and electro acupuncture, in which the current is passed down needles inserted in the skin, are accompanied by endopioid release into the cerebro-spinal fluid. It is also interesting to note that, to be maximally effective in various conditions, TENS needs to mimic closely ordinary manual acupuncture stimulation. The ideal wave form seems to be trains of high frequency impulses followed by electrical silence at a periodicity of two bursts per second. This is very similar to the nerve stimulation which occurs with rotation of an acupuncture needle between finger and thumb.

Long Term Cures

It is absolutely fascinating to be able to link the most modern scientific and medical research with a form of treatment originating in the China of five thousand years ago. Although much remains to be explained, there is no doubt that we are now well on the way to an understanding of acupuncture's mechanism of action, at any rate in the short term. A mystery still to be solved is how the effects of the acupuncture needle might continue long after it has been removed from the skin. It seems very likely that the inflammatory response to skin stimulation, which includes the release of various chemical mediators from damaged cells, lowers the response thresholds of local pain receptors. A state of hyperalgesia will then be caused in which the nerve cells would fire off in response to normally trivial stimulations for some time afterwards, thus keeping up a continual bombardment of the higher pain centres. Subsequent treatments at the same site would reinforce the effect. Even so, the response would be relatively short lived, lasting a matter of days only, and could not explain long term cures.

In certain cases an alteration of organ functioning, for some days or weeks, would allow a spontaneous healing process to ensue. For instance, if the secretion of acid from the stomach were consistently reduced for a period, an ulcer would have a chance to be healed by the stomach's normal reparative processes. Or if congestion round the opening of one of the nasal sinuses were reduced, the sinus would begin to drain freely and the chronic infection might then disappear. However, it is extremely difficult to use this kind of argument to explain the relief of many other kinds of illnesses, for instance, chronic neuralgias. In these some sort of permanent, or at least very long term, nervous system change must be taking place. To use our earlier analogy, we must postulate a rewiring of the control panel. This is not to say that there is an actual anatomical change in the brain or spinal cord, but merely that the balance of chemical and electrical activity between different pathways, which is both incredibly complex and exceedingly finely poised, is altered for long periods. We do not yet know how this might take place, but it would not be unique to acupuncture. After all, memory must represent this kind of change, albeit probably occurring in other parts of the brain than those involved in acupuncture stimulation.

Unknown Laws

The theories outlined in this chapter are certainly more than a little naïve, but probably represent at least a rough approximation of the changes which acupuncture brings about. Acupuncture suffers greatly from overstatement, but we have passed the stage where we can dismiss it as a form of hypnosis, or even charlatanism. There is well documented evidence that it is a highly effective form of therapy in appropriate cases. Preliminary research has provided an outline of its mode of action. There is now a clear need for further research as to the details of its physiological basis. This will not only lead to improvements in technique and, therefore, increases in therapeutic benefit, but also, I suggest, a greatly enhanced knowledge of the workings of our nervous systems. All this awaits further research for, as St Augustine is reputed to have said, 'There are no miracles, only unknown laws.'

Chapter 8

Case Reports

The following accounts of cases successfully treated with acupuncture illustrate the kinds of benefits which this form of treatment can bring about. They may be said to be typical instances of response to acupuncture, but it should not be assumed, by an intending patient, that their own complaint will behave in the same way. As stated many times in this book, there are enormous differences in the way individuals respond to this form of treatment and, even with the easiest condition to treat, the outcome cannot be guaranteed in all cases. Naturally, the best guidance as to the likely chances of improvement, as well as other aspects of therapy, will be obtained by discussing matters with the acupuncture practitioner.

Osteo-arthritis of the Hip
Mr A, a fifty-seven-year-old man, had had problems in the right hip for three-and-a-half years. This started with feelings of insecurity and progressed to pain, which became severe and, typically, radiated down to the knee. When he was first seen the pain was occurring every day, particularly on walking. Mr A could only manage 250 yards before the severity was such that he had to rest. To disguise this problem he had taken to pretending to look in shop windows and his progress down the High Street, when he went out from his

office to lunch, was punctuated by frequent episodes of 'window gazing'.

X-rays had previously confirmed the diagnosis of severe osteo-arthritis and he was under consideration for surgical treatment. He was not anxious to undergo surgery and for some months had been taking large quantities of pain killers and anti-inflammatory drugs to keep the symptoms under control. He had given up gardening, a hobby for many years, and viewed the future with some depression.

On clinical examination there was clear evidence of arthritis of the hip, with pain and restriction of movement of this joint. Mr A, only 5 foot 10 inches tall, weighted fifteen stone and his skinfold thickness indicated moderate obesity. Osteo-arthritis of the weightbearing joints is worsened by an excessive body weight, so a 1,000 calorie diet was recommended to bring this patient's weight to 12 stone 6 lbs, 'the desirable weight' according to tables published by Life Assurance companies.

Acupuncture points over the hip bone and sacrum were needled on five weekly occasions and then monthly. The anti-inflammatory drug, which he was taking, was considerably reduced in dosage after two months and walking distance had increased by then to half a mile. After four months Mr A had reduced his weight to twelve stone and was all but free of pain, except for a slight twinge in the hip when he moved it awkwardly. After six months I wrote to Mr A's general practitioner to say: 'you will be pleased to hear he has remained remarkably pain-free since I last wrote . . . he has now stopped all medication.'

It is important to emphasize that acupuncture cannot modify the underlying bony changes of osteo-arthritis, and there is a general tendency for this condition to worsen gradually as a person gets older. However, Mr A's case illustrates that it is often possible to obtain considerable symptomatic relief with acupuncture in this condition. Two further cases of osteo-arthritis will be described — concerning other commonly affected areas: the spine and knees.

★ ★ ★

Osteo-arthritis of the Lumbar Spine

Mr L was seventy-five years of age and had led a very active life since his retirement from work as a government scientist. He was a keen player of badminton and enjoyed walking and swimming. Like so many people, he had a little back pain over the years, following unusual exertion or strain, but in the previous twelve months the pain had become fairly constant and started to radiate down the left leg, and his general practitioner had diagnosed arthritic changes in the lumbar region of the spine.

On X-ray there was the characteristic narrowing of the joint spaces between adjacent vertebrae, and the spiky outgrowths of bone known as osteophytes. The changes were particularly severe between the second and third and the fourth and fifth lumbar vertebrae. In Mr L's case the problem was part of a wider picture, with mild arthritic changes also in the neck and knees.

Increasing interference with his hobbies finally prompted him to seek treatment and his family doctor advised acupuncture because the aspirin-like drugs he had been taking to relieve the pain were upsetting his stomach.

When he was seen first this patient had a fairly good range of spinal movements, but attempts to touch his toes caused a sharp pain in the back. Lying flat on his back, he could not raise his right leg, keeping the knee straight, to more than 45 degrees from the horizontal. As in so many similar cases, acupuncture points in the calf, buttock and back, were extremely tender to the touch. Needles were inserted at points on the side of the ankle, the outside of the calf, the buttock and in between and to the side of the relevant vertebrae — all on the affected side. In the week following the first treatment Mr L had considerably less pain and was able to abandon the walking stick he had required hitherto.

Two months later the pain had substantially disappeared and this patient was able to return to most of the activities he had previously been unable to carry out. He was given a good deal of advice about such things as sitting posture and the correct way to lift objects, which are matters of great importance to anybody with a bad back! Over the next three years this patient required further treatment at three to six monthly intervals to keep him as free from pain as possible and he simply telephoned when the symptoms started to get severe again and he knew that a treatment was overdue.

Osteo-arthritis of the Knees

Colonel H had been in the Indian Army many years before. In India he had played polo, but on his return took up golf and quickly became an addict. Now eighty-two, he had finally come to the realization that playing golf was impossible because of increasing pain and stiffness in both knees. A friend suggested acupuncture and, when I examined him, it was obvious that the arthritic changes in the knees were advanced. Both knees were swollen, there was a very limited range of movement and a creaking feeling, when a hand was put over the kneecap as the joint was extended. Other than that, Colonel H was in extremely good health and much frustrated by lack of mobility. The aim of treatment in this case was to at least provide some pain relief, although, clearly, in such an advanced case, the room for improvement was very small.

The first few treatments, involving insertion of needles just below and to the outside of the kneecaps and on the side of the leg near the head of the fine bone known as the fibula, passed without any problem. At first there was a little pain relief, but not much improvement in the amount of exercise that could be taken. Then, unfortunately, Colonel H got influenza and the pain in the knees returned with a vengeance. This 'breakthrough' of symptoms is quite common when some kind of intercurrent illness occurs during a course of treatment which may, up to that time, be producing a good result. After the Colonel had recovered, a further course of six treatments was carried out. At last there was a moderate improvement in walking distance and it was even possible for him to play nine holes of golf.

With great courage, typical of someone of his background, and realizing that weightbearing exercise would in future be very difficult, Colonel H decided to take up swimming to keep fit. Soon after the completion of the last course of treatment he moved from the area but wrote a little later, saying that the pain relief was continuing.

Post Herpetic Neuralgia

One of the most difficult, painful conditions which any doctor is called upon to treat is that of post herpetic neuralgia: the pain which arises following 'shingles', which is infection of the skin and nerves by the virus known as herpes zoster. In fact, to describe the condition simply as pain is inaccurate. It consists also of burning or itching sensations in the distribution of the affected nerves, usually on the chest or abdomen and some-times on the side of the face. The chances of developing neuralgia after an attack of shingles are much higher in the elderly and there is evidence to show that if the initial acute infection is inadequately treated these distressing sequelae are also more likely.

A wide variety of methods has been used to alleviate the discomfort which is caused, ranging from drugs to injection of nerves or even section of parts of the spinal cord. Mrs T had had a moderately severe attack of shingles, affecting the left side of the chest, three years previously. The rash cleared fairly quickly, but even many months afterwards it was possible to see where it had been because of a residue of depig-mentation in the skin of the affected area. After the initial pain of the infection there was a period of about one year free from symptoms, but then severe pain had recurred, as well as ten-derness and, during the worst time, Mrs T could not even bear the touch of clothing on her back.

A number of treatments had already been tried, without effect, and whilst simple painkillers had initially provided relief, the problem had worsened until strong morphine-like drugs were being taken in increasing doses, with a correspon-ding risk of addiction. The lack of response led to this patient becoming very depressed and anti-depressant medication was required. This in turn led to drowsiness during the day, com-pounded by lack of sleep at night due to pain, which was interfering with everyday activities including car driving.

All in all, things seemed to be going from bad to worse and

the patient was referred to the hospital pain relief clinic for consideration of more heroic therapies. Injections of the nerves running between the ribs with local anaesthetic solution provided only short term relief. The next thing tried was transcutaneous electrical nerve stimulation (TENS), placing electrodes at the front and back and passing a small current between. This also produced some improvement and since this often suggests that acupuncture will be beneficial, possibly for a longer period, this form of treatment was finally tried. A chain of points running along the backbone was stimulated and electro-acupuncture was administered to points on the feet, leg and side of the chest.

The unpleasant tingling sensation which accompanied the pain was immediately abolished and did not return. Each weekly treatment was followed by two to four days of complete pain relief and, finally, the addition of a small night time dose of an anti-convulsant drug, to reduce the 'irritability' of the nervous system, completed the cure, allowing the withdrawal of the other painkilling medication.

This case illustrates the need for acupuncture to be considered as one of the many treatment modalities which can be offered in the modern medical approach to a condition resistant to conventional treatment alone.

Trigeminal Neuralgia

Trigeminal neuralgia is another most unpleasant painful condition, often very hard to treat. It is manifest as a severe lancinating pain in the side of the face, of unknown cause. Mr N had suffered from this for about two years and was being treated with Tegretol, a drug often used for this condition, which provided partial relief but caused such severe side-effects in the high doses necessary that his life was as much affected by the treatment as it had been by the disease. Mr N was a keen skier and found the combination of fatigue and a cold draught on the side of his face a very potent stimulus in causing an attack of the pain. For this reason and because of disturbances of balance caused by his drug therapy, he had largely given up his hobby.

During a business trip to the Far East he was treated by a traditional Chinese acupuncturist, with the result that he returned to the United Kingdom completely free of pain and off all medication. The Chinese practitioner had inserted needles into the side of the face and into a point which is often used for a variety of conditions: the 'Ho Ku' point between the thumb and first finger on the back of the hand. The treatment which had been given abroad was standard acupuncture, utilizing a combination of points which would be treated for this condition also in the West.

Follow-up treatments given initially every few weeks and then only when the pain threatened to recur prevented the neuralgia from coming back. This patient learned to treat himself and, in future, always took a number of acupuncture needles with him when he went on a skiing holiday.

Eczema

Mr H, a twenty-seven-year-old plumber, had suffered from eczema since he was a child. Like other patients with an allergic tendency, he also used to get hay fever during the spring and early summer and was liable to become wheezy when he took severe exercise or had an infection of the upper airways, such as a cold. The respiratory manifestations of his allergy were gradually improving, but the eczema remained extremely troublesome, particularly in the hot weather; itching causing general distraction during the day and loss of sleep at night. Contact with oils and substances used for caulking during his work increased the inflammation and he was seriously considering a change of occupation.

Mr H was being seen by the dermatologist at the local hospital and was being treated with local applications, as well as sleeping tablets and antihistamine drugs to reduce the irritation. Even a short course of steroid tablets, only given in the worst cases, produced only partial relief and was then stopped because of the risk of developing severe side-effects with prolonged use. The condition always cleared up during Mr T's summer holiday if he went to the seaside and swam and bathed a lot but, short of becoming a tropical beachcomber, this was hardly a practical, long-term solution!

Results with acupuncture in skin conditions can be very variable, but in this patient's case the treatment produced an excellent result, albeit a gradual one. Needling of points on the hands, legs and feet led to a reduction of itching within three weeks, and by one month both arms and legs were clearly less inflamed. Mr T was then seen approximately monthly on four occasions, at the end of which time the rash had changed in character, being more punctate and less generalized, with a considerable reduction in scaliness. He was taking much less antihistamine and hypnotic medication since the itching was less troublesome. He was seen three times more in total, showing a continued substantial improvement

Post Traumatic Neuralgia

Occasionally an injury, in which nerves are involved, does not heal normally but gives rise to severe neuralgic pains for months or years afterwards. This can even happen when only the fine nerves in the skin seem to have been involved; for example, when a traumatic or operative scar is painful after apparently healing.

Miss M was a twenty-one-year-old secretary, who sustained a laceration to the left cheek two years previously. An X-ray showed no bony injury and the small cut was stitched normally. In the ensuing months the site became painful and swelled up again on several occasions. It was surgically re-explored, but no abnormality was found. Despite this, the scar itself was very painful and there was an aching in front of the ear, radiating into the teeth and eye on that side. The pain occurred once or twice every fortnight and usually lasted one or two days, but could last for up to four days. It was worsened by cold, but not by chewing (a feature which, if present, would have suggested a problem with the teeth or with the joint of the jaw).

On examination there was nothing abnormal to find, except a slightly swollen one-inch scar tender to the touch, over the cheek bone. Miss M was treated by inserting needles into points on the face above and below the scar and underneath the nose. After the first treatment there was a small improvement and, by the third, the pain was about 25 per cent less. Because of the slowness of the response, two further points, at the lower margin of the jaw on the affected side, were added. In the ensuing two weeks there was no pain at all and, apart from occasional twinges, this was the situation over the next nine months. At this time Miss. M. was discharged with a caution to contact me again for treatment if the pain returned.

Obesity

The use of acupuncture to treat obesity and addiction to cigarettes is sometimes dismissed by medical practitioners as trivial but, in my opinion, fulfils a very important medical function, since over-eating and smoking are causes of a very great deal of ill health in our community. The technique for treating these cases has undergone a change in recent years; most acupuncture practitioners now using an indwelling 'press needle' held in place in the ear for days or weeks. There is a slightly greater risk of infection from these needles, but the results are very encouraging. The following two cases illustrate the benefits which may be obtained.

Mrs J, a pleasant lady from Lancashire, aged thirty-eight, had had two children. She had put on a good deal of weight when carrying these, but had lost it when she stopped breast feeding. The youngest child was three years of age, and over the previous twelve months the patient's body-weight had started to rise again. There was no obvious reason for this; not much stress and no sign of a hormonal or other medical cause of the problem; but Mrs J simply found it extremely difficult to stick to diets because of her love of cooking and eating good food.

There seems no doubt that people are, by birth, either lucky or unlucky in this respect. Many people put on large amounts of body weight with a food intake which would hardly keep body and soul together in other individuals.

In Mrs J's case, after the failure of a session at *Weight Watchers*, acupuncture was suggested by a relative, and her general practitioner readily agreed. When she was first seen her weight was 14 stone 2 lbs and her height 5 foot 5 inches. The thickness of the skin at the back of the arm (a reliable guide to the presence of subcutaneous fat) was 3.7 cm. Obese people are rather more liable to a raised blood pressure, but this was normal in Mrs J's case. Following discussion of the problem, a tiny press needle was placed in the appropriate point of the right ear (because the patient habitually slept with the left side of her head against the pillow). Insertion of the press needle was completely painless, and it was held in place with a small piece of sticking plaster. Mrs J was given a diet sheet and asked to return in a fortnight for a review of her case.

When she came back she was clearly delighted with the results. The diet was similar to others she had tried previously but, in this case, the acupuncture treatment seemed to act as if turning off a tap: she had no desire to eat more than the small amount of food allowed in her régime. The press needle had, in fact, fallen out after ten days, which is to be expected, but the diminished appetite drive was continuing. The duration of effect of this treatment is often many weeks and, in any case, once the appetite is re-educated with a little help from acupuncture, most patients are able to continue unassisted.

The rate of relapse in treating overweight patients is depressingly high when they are seen again months or even years later. However, the treatment can easily be repeated and the results with acupuncture seem at least as good as with other methods of reducing the appetite. Also, the treatment is associated with far fewer side-effects than, say, appetite suppressing drugs.

Smoking

Mr D, at forty-three, had risen to become the Managing Director of the company he worked for. He worked hard in a job that imposed a good deal of stress upon him. He had smoked since he was sixteen years old and was, currently, on thirty a day. He was well aware of the health risks, being an intelligent person and, a few years ago, had swopped to a low-tar brand of cigarette when these became available. He was still concerned about his health, however, although the cost of smoking was relatively unimportant to him.

On examination, Mr D's chest was, in fact, clear and a measurement of 'peak expiratory flow rate' (a measure of the speed with which air can be expelled from the lungs) was normal. This last can be a useful indication of effects on the lungs from chronic smoking. The measurement is also reduced in cases of bronchitis and asthma. Actually even after years of heavy smoking there may be little sign of damage to the lungs, but there is an increased risk of developing numerous diseases later in life.

The point indicated for treatment of cigarette addiction, on the lobe of the ear, was tender on the left hand side when touched gently with the shaft of an acupuncture needle. This is often the case and is a guide to localization of the point. A press needle was placed into position and held with a piece of sticking plaster, as in the previous case. Mr D was asked to stop smoking cigarettes immediately; experience having shown that gradual reduction is of no value whatsoever. He was told that, if the craving for a cigarette became intense, the treatment's effect could be reinforced by gripping the press needle and the lobe of the ear between finger and thumb and squeezing gently. He was very interested in the possible mechanism of action and it was explained that insertion of a needle into the appropriate ear point probably resulted in release of certain chemicals in the brain (called endorphins) which substituted for similar release of chemicals caused by smoking cigarettes. One month after the treatment I received a letter from the patient, which said: 'Treatment a complete success, have not touched a cigarette since . . .'

Migraine
Selection of the appropriate case of migraine to present, in this list of reports, has proved extremely difficult because of the large number treated. It is a very distressing condition for the patient but, fortunately, one which is relatively easy to treat with acupuncture. Each case is slightly different, with diffe-

rent predisposing factors such as worry, diet, consumption of alcohol and so on, and different combinations of pain, visual disturbances, tingling and perhaps even paralysis. Most patients seen by the acupuncturist seem to be adults, but migraine does occur in children and the following is a case point.

Master K had suffered from migraine symptoms since the age of five, but they had only been recognized as migraine over the last three years. This is a common story in children, whose attacks of 'biliousness' are often ascribed to over-eating, expecially when they follow a party or other treat. In fact, it is often the nervous excitement of the party environment which causes the problem not the excessive consumption of food!

This boy complained of pain in the head, occurring on either side, but never on both sides at once. The pain was felt in the region of the eye and running round to the temple, but never in the forehead or back of the head. Like many migraine sufferers, Master K could tell when he was about to have an attack because he felt tired and out of sorts. A fully developed episode would result in nausea and then vomiting. Luckily, in his case, there was no neurological disturbance, such as tingling in fingers, and nor were there visual symptoms, such as the appearance of bright sparkling lights or losses of part of the visual field.

Master K was aged thirteen when I saw him first and his parents were extremely concerned that his career at school was being adversely affected by his headaches. They rarely occurred during vacation periods, but times of stress at school often led to problems. Thus attacks might occur just before examinations or on the school's sports day. He had been treated with a large variety of medications, including tran-quillizers and pain killing drugs specific for migraine. There seemed little doubt that the symptoms were getting steadily worse and, with increasing pressure due to the need to study harder as he got older, the boy's outlook seemed depressing.

Paediatric patients do not much like needles! Accordingly, I treated this patient with a light spiked hammer, tapping the appropriate points twenty or thirty times until a satisfactory skin reaction was obtained. The points chosen were those on the top of the feet, the tops of the shoulders and behind the ears. After three such treatments the headaches were continuing unabated and there was a clear need to alter the choice of points. A change to points on the side of the head on a level with the eyes and above and behind the tips of the ear lobes, proved rapidly successful. It was possible to reduce the medication progressively as the frequency and severity of attacks abated. Master K was taught how to massage the same points when he experienced the aura which usually preceded an attack. By doing so he was able to abort several attacks before they actually occurred.

This patient was seen off and on for three years. Treatments every four to six months kept him free of attacks and he returned each time he felt mild warnings that the problem might be recurring. At the end of this time no further treatments were necessary, probably in part due to the normal change which had occurred by then, from schoolboy into mature young man.

Rheumatoid Arthritis

The condition of rheumatoid arthritis is extremely interesting from a medical and scientific point of view. The way in which it is caused is extremely complicated and probably involves alterations to the body's immunological mechanisms. There is some evidence that acupuncture, given very early in the disease, can modify the development of it. However, the case I would like to describe, concerns a patient who had had the problems for very many years and in whom symptomatic relief only was possible; although this was most worthwhile from the point of view of relief of suffering.

Mrs E was seventy-two years old and had suffered from rheumatoid arthritis since she was about fifty. Typically, it flitted from joint to joint, affecting, in turn, wrists, ankles, knees, elbows and fingers. Over the years she had had a variety of treatments. Many drugs had been tried, including the old and trusted remedies of aspirin and indomethacin, as well as many of the newer non-steroidal anti-inflammatory drugs, corticosteroids and even injections of gold. This last drug offers the chance of modifying the underlying disease process in some way, and not just giving symptomatic relief, but is associated with a severe risk of side-effects which entails very careful monitoring of the condition of any patient receiving it.

When I saw Mrs E her arthritis had largely burnt out. She was in good general health, and no longer suffered from the lassitude and anaemia she had been affected by when the arthritis was in an active phase. The right elbow joint was, however, still inflamed and hot to the touch, although this was settling gradually. As a result of the many successive attacks of inflammation there was considerable residual deformity and reduction in range of movement of the joints. Mrs E had been keen on knitting all through her life and had produced many pairs of gloves, scarves and jerseys for her grandchildren. Now, unfortunately, because of the degree of muscle wasting and deformity in the hands and wrists this was no longer possible. Despite a good deal of sympathetic support from her husband, this patient had become very depressed in recent months and feared that, in due course, she would become completely crippled. Fortunately it was possible to explain that this was not likely to be the case and that clearly after so many years, the arthritis was now quietening down and that, with the help of acupuncture, a good deal of symptomatic relief might be provided which would make life much more tolerable.

The most severely affected joints were concentrated on first. Mrs E had a good deal of pain and stiffness in the right knee, the left ankle and the joints of many of her fingers on both hands. She embarked upon a course of treatments lasting about two months. On each occasion the relevant points close to the affected joints were treated either with the needles or with a 'star hammer'. At the same time she was given advice about exercise, rest, warm bathing and other physical treatments which would help reduce the disability and the level of symptoms. In such a long-standing condition, it was to be expected that improvement would be gradual. However, benefit occurred steadily and, at the end of the initial course of therapy, Mrs E was very much better than previously. During this period the acute inflammation of the elbow had subsided, and the constant encouragement and emphasis on the positive aspects of her illness had altered Mrs E's outlook so that she was much more optimistic about the future. Over the ensuing months and years the treatment was repeated at intervals, the patient herself deciding when a session to reinforce the effect was necessary. No more acute flare-ups of the arthritic condition occurred.

★ ★ ★

Prolapsed Intervertebral Disc

Mr F, thirty-six years of age, was a jobbing gardener. When I saw him first he was very concerned about the possible need to give up his occupation because of a bad back. The history was that he had suffered a prolapsed intervertebral disc about three months previously and had spent a spell in hospital as a result. In this condition, the gristle-like material between adjacent vertebrae extrudes into the space around the spinal nerves. There is acute pain in the back as a result and, if the disc actually presses on the nerves, a radiating discomfort down the course of the nerves in the leg and buttock and, possibly, even disturbances of bladder and bowel functions.

Mr F was spared this last problem, but did have severe pain along the course of the sciatic nerve on the left-hand side, together with tingling and numbness on the outside of the calf and in the foot. This had persisted despite a period of enforced bed rest and was little affected by painkilling drugs. When asked to bend his back in various directions, Mr F could almost touch his toes, but the last few inches of flexion were accompanied by quite severe pain. Rotation of the spine to the left and right was pain free and could be accomplished to the normal extent. Lying flat on his back on the couch, he could raise the right leg, with the knee straight, perpendicularly above the couch. On the left-hand side, however, the leg could only be raised to make an angle of 60 degrees with the horizontal. All the reflexes in the lower limbs were equally active and sensation in the skin of the leg and foot was unchanged.

In a case of this kind, particularly with somebody who has an active, physical job, advice as to the best method of lifting and carrying objects, as well as the most comfortable sitting position, is critically important. A long time was spent in explaining the 'ins and outs' of this and then treatment was given to points on the side of the left ankle, on the side of the calf, on the buttock and in the middle of the spine, as well as to the side of it, at the affected level. Mr F was seen a week later, when the pain in the back was unchanged, but the radiating pain down the left leg had diminished and the pins and needles in the foot and calf had entirely gone. A small adjustment was made to the treatment and the patient returned in a further week. Remarkably, there had been almost no pain at all in the intervening seven days, and when the spinal movement and straight leg raising tests were repeated, these were found to be perfectly normal. The treatment was repeated twice more for good measure at two and three weekly intervals and, at the end of this time, Mr F had been completely free of pain except for very occasional twinges following heavy manual work. He was reviewed after six weeks and again three months later, when the story was unchanged.

Frozen Shoulder

Some joints in the body are particularly easy to treat with acupuncture. Others, such as the shoulder, are more resistant. This case describes a sixty-four-year-old housewife, who injured her shoulder during a spring cleaning session. Her general practitioner diagnosed a soft tissue strain, advised rest and prescribed simple painkillers. The condition did not resolve over the next few months and the doctor then gave a local injection of analgesic and steroid solution to try to speed up healing. There was a temporary improvement, but the shoulder soon became stiff and painful again. It did not get better at all during the ensuing six months and, indeed, if anything, was slightly worse. There was then clear limitation of movement and the diagnosis of 'frozen shoulder' was made.

This condition can be extremely chronic and the danger is that, because of pain, the patient restricts the movement of the joint, so losing muscle power and making eventual return to full mobility much more difficult. When I saw Mrs L for the first time, she was clearly 'guarding' her shoulder; preventing it from being jolted as she undressed. It was tender to the touch in several areas at the front and on the top. It was not obviously swollen, but could not be moved beyond a very limited range without considerable pain. Mrs L had given up taking painkillers because they produced only very temporary relief and, beyond holding a hot water bottle against the joint at night, was doing nothing for the condition at all.

A careful examination of the skin and underlying tissues showed that many of the acupuncture points in the area were extremely tender. These points were first massaged again until tenderness eventually went. I explained that, even with acupuncture, the condition might take a long time to resolve. At the same time I suggested gentle swinging exercises to reduce the stiffness and help to ensure that, eventually, a full range of movement would be possible. One week later the patient returned. She had felt much better for three days but then, following a bout of ironing, the pain had returned to its previous level. Nonetheless, on examination, the local acupuncture points were much less painful to the touch. The same points were treated and a week later Mrs L returned again. This time, there had been no response whatsoever to treatment and the patient was most disappointed. On enquiry, it transpired that she had had a sore throat during this period and she could be reassured that the seeming lack of response might well have been due to this inter-current illness.

If it had not been for this, I might well have changed the points to an alternative combination, but in the event decided to treat the same points yet again. In all, Mrs L had four more treatments and progress was then slow but steady. At the end of the course of acupuncture she was able to move her arm without pain, although the range of movement was still somewhat restricted. I explained that the solution to this was in her own hands and that, provided the exercises were maintained, full movement of the shoulder joint could be expected to return over a period of months.

★ ★ ★

Hay Fever

Mr T was a nineteen-year-old university student studying economics. He had had severe hay fever for twelve years, a problem recurring every spring and disappearing in the middle of the summer when the pollen count returned to low levels. During the pollen season his life was made a misery by sneezing, running eyes and a sore throat. In fact pollen was not the only problem. Skin tests a few years previously had shown strong reactions to a variety of allergens including house dust, and animal fur and skin. Amongst the medical treatments which had been tried were antihistamine tablets (which made him feel very drowsy), a corticosteroid nasal spray, a series of desensitizing injections, and inhalation of the anti-allergic drug known as Intal.

Examination by the ENT surgeons had shown that Mr T had rather narrow nostrils as well as a number of small out-growths of the nasal mucous membrane known as polyps. These had been removed surgically, but overall the condition had been little changed. Apart from this, Mr T was in very good health. He was a keen sportsman, playing squash in the winter and tennis in the summer. Of course the hay fever interfered with the tennis to some extent. In fact when his eyes were running badly he sometimes had difficulty in seeing the ball! Mr T had heard about acupuncture from a friend who had been successfully treated by another practitioner.

In the case of hay fever and other ear, nose and throat afflic-tions, an important chain of points lies on the 'Large Intestine meridian' which runs up from the back of the hand over the side of the elbow on to the neck and terminates, having crossed the mid-line, at the side of the nose.

The large doses of antihistamine that Mr T was taking seemed to be providing little benefit and so were drastically reduced, with an immediate improvement in alertness during the day. Points on the above channel were treated both locally around the nose and upper lip and at a distance from the affected area on the top of the hands. Mr T felt slightly faint after this and, although this reaction is slightly more common in young men and may be considered normal, it was taken as an indication that the treatment had been too vigorous. Often, as explained elsewhere in this book, an acupuncture treatment which is carried out too strongly is less effective than a more moderate one. This indeed seemed to be the case for Mr T who returned a week after this treatment, saying that although he had been very much better for a while, the improvement starting within twenty-four hours, the symptoms returned on the following day. Even so, a walk in the country during the week had not produced the profuse nasal discharge and feeling of stuffiness that would normally have been expected.

From then on the course of the improvement was very smooth. Mr T required three more treatments at fortnightly intervals, by the end of which time the symptoms had stopped completely. A month after this the pollen season was over and I advised the patient to return for a brief course of acupuncture treatment early next spring. This he did, and this prevented the symptoms showing at all that year.

In choosing cases treated by acupuncture to present here, I have purposely selected those in whom beneficial results occurred. This is not to say, of course, that benefit occurs in every case, but it shows what can be achieved. Treatment failures are edifying and important for the practitioner, because by studying them he may learn how to reduce their frequency in future. On the other hand, it is obviously the results of a successful outcome which will be of most interest to an intending patient. As stated several times before, the chances of success vary considerably from one condition to another, as well as from one patient to another, and the best guide to this will be a discussion of one's own particular complaint with the acupuncturist.

Index